T0182111

Biology and Management of Unusual Plasma Cell Dyscrasias

Todd M. Zimmerman · Shaji K. Kumar
Editors

Biology and Management of Unusual Plasma Cell Dyscrasias

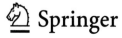

Editors
Todd M. Zimmerman, MD
Section of Hematology/Oncology
The University of Chicago
Chicago, IL, USA

Shaji K. Kumar, MD
Division of Hematology,
  Department of Medicine
Mayo Clinic
Rochester, MN, USA

ISBN 978-1-4939-7926-4   ISBN 978-1-4419-6848-7   (eBook)
DOI 10.1007/978-1-4419-6848-7

© Springer Science+Business Media New York 2017
Softcover reprint of the hardcover 1st edition 2016
This work is subject to copyright. All rights are reserved by the Publisher, whether the whole or part of the material is concerned, specifically the rights of translation, reprinting, reuse of illustrations, recitation, broadcasting, reproduction on microfilms or in any other physical way, and transmission or information storage and retrieval, electronic adaptation, computer software, or by similar or dissimilar methodology now known or hereafter developed.
The use of general descriptive names, registered names, trademarks, service marks, etc. in this publication does not imply, even in the absence of a specific statement, that such names are exempt from the relevant protective laws and regulations and therefore free for general use.
The publisher, the authors and the editors are safe to assume that the advice and information in this book are believed to be true and accurate at the date of publication. Neither the publisher nor the authors or the editors give a warranty, express or implied, with respect to the material contained herein or for any errors or omissions that may have been made.

Printed on acid-free paper

This Springer imprint is published by Springer Nature
The registered company is Springer Science+Business Media LLC New York

Preface

The past decade has witnessed unprecedented advances in the understanding of monoclonal gammopathies, driven both by the availability of new therapeutic agents as well as a better understanding of the biology of plasma cell disorders. While the focus in the field has been on multiple myeloma, its diagnosis, risk stratification, and therapies, we have also made significant progress in understanding the less common monoclonal gammopathies. Many of the lessons that we have learned in the context of multiple myeloma have widespread application for the less common plasma cell disorders. With testing for monoclonal proteins becoming more commonplace and the introduction of serum free light chain assay, allowing for detection of monoclonal proteins previously missed on traditional serum protein electrophoresis, monoclonal gammopathy and associated disorders are increasingly being diagnosed.

While there are numerous publications in the area of multiple myeloma, very few review articles and book chapters are dedicated to the less common plasma cell disorders. This is a rapidly expanding area with more sensitive diagnostic technology, such as mass spectrometry, allowing us to identify small amounts of protein hitherto not appreciated by the conventional diagnostic assays. Other advances in technology, such as next-generation sequencing as well as highly sensitive multiparameter flow cytometry, have contributed to our ability to detect and diagnose these rare plasma cell disorders. Not only has the ability to detect the small plasma cell clones been enhanced through these technologies, we have also become more aware of the various disease associations and the potential contribution of the monoclonal protein to disease manifestations. This is particularly relevant in the context of many uncommon renal disorders that were not previously associated with monoclonal proteins.

We have brought together many of the renowned experts in this field with the intent of developing a state-of-the-art reference that will allow clinicians and scientists to get a better understanding of these uncommon disorders. We have dedicated individual chapters to each of these disorders, with each chapters outlining what is currently known about the pathophysiology of these disorders as well as the common treatment approaches. We hope that the information in this book will not only help guide management of the patient in the clinic, but also form the basis for future studies related to these disorders. We sincerely hope that you will find this book to be a great addition to the literature in the field and a constant guide in your daily practice.

Chicago, USA   Todd M. Zimmerman, MD
Rochester, USA   Shaji K. Kumar, MD

Contents

Contributors

Stephen M. Ansell, MD, PhD Division of Hematology, Department of Medicine, Mayo Clinic, Rochester, MN, USA

Francis K. Buadi, MB, ChB Division of Hematology, Department of Medicine, Mayo Clinic, Rochester, MN, USA

Anita D'Souza, MD, MS Department of Medicine, Medical College of Wisconsin, Milwaukee, WI, USA

Angela Dispenzieri, MD Division of Hematology, Department of Medicine, Mayo Clinic, Rochester, MN, USA

Wilson I. Gonsalves, MD Division of Hematology, Department of Medicine, Mayo Clinic, Rochester, MN, USA

Vinay Gupta, MD Division of Hematology, Department of Medicine, Mayo Clinic, Rochester, MN, USA

Amara S. Hussain, MD Department of Medicine, Medical College of Wisconsin, Milwaukee, WI, USA

Prashant Kapoor, MD Division of Hematology, Department of Medicine, Mayo Clinic, Rochester, MN, USA

Shaji K. Kumar, MD Division of Hematology, Department of Medicine, Mayo Clinic, Rochester, MN, USA

Nelson Leung, MD Departments of Nephrology and Hypertension, Hematology, Mayo Clinic, Rochester, MN, USA

Samih H. Nasr, MD Department of Laboratory Medicine and Pathology, Mayo Clinic, Rochester, MN, USA

Nidhi Tandon, MD Division of Hematology, Department of Medicine, Mayo Clinic, Rochester, MN, USA

Todd M. Zimmerman, MD Section of Hematology/Oncology, The University of Chicago, Chicago, IL, USA

Abbreviations

Ang 2	Angiopoietin 2
ASCT	Autologous stem cell transplant
C3 GN	C3 Monoclonal associated glomerulonephritis
HCDD	Heavy chain deposition disease
HMVECs	Human microvascular endothelial cells
ITG	Immunotactoid glomerulonephropathy (ITG)
IVIG	Intravenous immunoglobulin
LCDD	Light chain deposition disease
LHCDD	Mixed light and heavy chain deposition disease
MGUS	Monoclonal gammopathy of undetermined significance
PGNMID	Proliferative glomerulonephritis with monoclonal IgG deposits
SCLS	Systemic capillary leak syndrome
SNP	Single nucleotide polymorphism
VEGF	Vascular endothelial growth factor

Chapter 1
Plasma Cell Leukemia

Wilson I. Gonsalves, MD and Shaji K. Kumar, MD

Introduction

Plasma cell dyscrasias account for roughly 10 % of all hematologic malignancies [1]. There is a wide spectrum of plasma cell neoplasms that includes monoclonal gammopathy of undetermined significance (MGUS), smoldering myeloma (SMM), multiple myeloma (MM), and plasma cell leukemia (PCL) in the order of increasing malignant potential and aggressiveness. While circulating clonal plasma cells (PCs) can be seen in all stages including MGUS, they generally make up only a small fraction of the peripheral blood cells, with most of the clonal PCs are limited to the bone marrow. PCL on the other hand is characterized by the presence of a significant number of circulating clonal PCs. The first

W.I. Gonsalves, MD (✉) · S.K. Kumar, MD
Division of Hematology, Department of Medicine, Mayo Clinic, 200 First Street SW, Rochester, MN 55905, USA
e-mail: gonsalves.wilson@mayo.edu

S.K. Kumar, MD
e-mail: kumar.shaji@mayo.edu

© Springer Science+Business Media New York 2017
T.M. Zimmerman and S.K. Kumar (eds.),
Biology and Management of Unusual Plasma Cell Dyscrasias,
DOI 10.1007/978-1-4419-6848-7_1

case of PCL was described in 1906 by Gluzinski and Reichenstein [2]. However, it was not until 1974 that Kyle et al. defined it as the presence of more than 20 % PCs in the peripheral blood or an absolute PC count in the peripheral blood of greater than 2.0×10^9 cells/L [3, 4]. Primary PCL (pPCL) refers to those cases that originate de novo with no prior history of MM, whereas secondary PCL (sPCL) refers to cases where patients with a prior history of MM develop a leukemic phase of their MM.

Epidemiology

PCL is relatively rare and accounts for less than 5 % of all plasma cell neoplasms. In the United States, PCL has been estimated to have an incidence of 0.04–0.05/100,000 [5]. pPCL accounts for majority of the PCL cases (60–70 %) and sPCL being the remainder of cases [6]. sPCL occurs as a progressive event of the disease in 1–4 % of patients with MM [5]. However, with the improvement in survival experienced by patients with MM, many are living long enough to have their MM transform into sPCL [5, 7]. The median time for MM to evolve into sPCL has been reported as 21 months [8]; however, this is likely increasing given the incorporation of novel agent therapies in the upfront management of MM that have provided longer durations of disease control.

Clinical Characteristics

Given the lack of prospective clinical data, most information regarding the clinical presentation of pPCL and sPCL is derived from retrospective single-institution series [8–15]. Patients with pPCL tend to be younger in age with the median age of diagnosis of 55 years compared with 71 years in MM and sPCL [8]. pPCL may be more prevalent in African Americans than Caucasians or Asian–Pacific Islanders [16]. Patients with pPCL tend to have a higher predisposition to developing extramedullary disease such as hepatomegaly, splenomegaly, lymphadenopathy, pleural effusions, neurological deficits secondary to central nervous system involvement, and soft tissue plasmacytomas [15]. They also tend to have more light chain-only secreting disease and higher amounts of bone marrow involvement leading to anemia and thrombocytopenia [7, 11]. pPCL patients are more likely to present with elevated LDH, increased β2-microglobulin, renal insufficiency, and hypercalcemia [14, 17]. However, extensive lytic bone lesions are more common in patients with MM and sPCL [8]; the latter likely because it is the terminal stage of preexistent MM. Extramedullary involvement is less common in sPCL than pPCL [8, 9]. Finally, even though patients with sPCL often present with renal insufficiency, it is still more common in pPCL than sPCL [16].

Pathological Characteristics

Morphology

The morphology of clonal PCs present in the bone marrow core biopsy and aspirate of patients with either pPCL or sPCL can be similar to those seen in MM but at times may appear more immature or plasmablastic. The infiltration of the clonal PCs is diffuse and typically disrupts normal hematopoiesis [8, 18]. In most patients with pPCL or sPCL, the peripheral blood typically has a leuko-erythroblastic picture [8, 18]. Identification of the sine qua non circulating clonal PCs in the peripheral blood is difficult by light microscopy alone as it is hard to differentiate them from circulating clonal lymphocytes and typically warrants immunophenotypic analysis via flow cytometry.

Immunophenotype

There are several similarities and differences between the immunophenotype markers present on the clonal PCs found in patients with pPCL, sPCL, and MM. Even though the clonal PCs in both MM and the different forms of PCL are positive for CD38 and CD138, there is progressive decrease in the level of CD38 expression in the clonal PCs obtained from PCL compared with

MM reflecting a more immature phenotype in the former [19]. PCs from patients with either forms of PCL are less likely to express CD9, CD56, CD71, CD117, and HLA-DR; however, they are more likely to express CD20, CD45, CD19, CD27, and CD23 [11, 20–22]. When comparing pPCL and sPCL against each other, CD28 and CD56 are more likely to be present on the clonal PCs obtained from patients with sPCL and have been linked to higher proliferation index and rate of disease progression [20].

Proliferative Index

Clonal PCs cells in pPCL are different from those in MM in terms of their predominant cell cycle phase, with the former showing a higher percentage of PCs in S-phase implicating a higher proliferative index [11].

Molecular Cytogenetics

Most patients with either pPCL tend to have non-hyperdiploid karyotypes (hypodiploid or diploid) in contrast to MM where half of new patients are hyperdiploid [8, 23]. The various types of IgH (14q32) translocations by FISH analysis are present in more than 80 % of both forms of PCL. The most prevalent IgH translocation in pPCL is t(11;14) [24]. The incidence of t(4;14) and t(14;16) in pPCL and sPCL is also higher than in newly diagnosed MM [24, 25]. Finally, the presence of del(13q), del(17p), del(1p21), ampl (1q21) or CKS1B overexpression and MYC translocations or amplifications is very common in both pPCL and sPCL [8, 24–26]. All of these secondary events have been associated with a trend toward inferior OS in pPCL and sPCL.

Molecular Genetics

Activating mutations of K-RAS or N-RAS at codons 12, 13, or 61 are found in highest frequency in patients with pPCL but can also be detected in patients with sPCL as well as MM and have been associated with poor OS [8, 27, 28]. There is also a relatively higher incidence of PTEN deletion resulting in Akt activation in the clonal PCs from patients with PCL compared with MM suggesting its role as a secondary event possibly in the transition from MM to PCL [29]. pPCL patients treated on the Total Therapy protocols who had high-risk signatures by the GEP-70 and GEP-80 models (44 and 31 %) were found to differentially express 203 different genes. Some of these genes included CD14 (cell membrane LPS receptor), TNF receptor-associated factor 2, and chemokine C–C motif ligand suggesting the possibility of a myeloid differentiation of plasma cells during leukemic development [17]. Egan et al. [30] conducted whole-genome sequencing in serial samples from a single patient through different time points in their clinical course, including at the time of development of sPCL which identified various unique single nucleotide variants (SNVs) in the following genes during the sPCL phase: *RB1, TNN, TUBB8, ZKSCAN3*, and *ZNF521*.

Diagnostic Testing

Patients suspected of having either form of PCL must undergo a detailed medical history and physical examination. This should be accompanied by a comprehensive evaluation of their blood through the following tests: complete blood count with differential, peripheral blood smear, peripheral blood flow cytometry, BUN, creatinine, liver enzymes, bilirubin, alkaline phosphatase, total protein, CRP, LDH, electrolyte panel, uric acid, β-2-microglobulin, albumin, serum protein electrophoresis with immunofixation, and serum free light chain analysis. They should also undergo a 24-h urine collection for electrophoresis, immunofixation, and total protein assessment. All patients require a bone marrow biopsy and aspirate to assess for morphology, immunophenotyping, and cytogenetic analysis by FISH focused on del(17p13), del(13q), del(1p21), ampl(1q21), t(11;14), t(4;14), t(14;20), and t(14;16). Gene expression profiling is not universally available at all facilities but can be performed for further risk stratification. Finally, whole-body imaging with either a whole-body MRI, CT, or [18] F-FDG-PET/CT to assess for not only bony lytic lesions but also extramedullary involvement is necessary.

Trends in Reported Survival Outcomes

The survival of patients with pPCL is poor compared with newly diagnosed MM but still longer than patients with sPCL. An analysis of the SEER database evaluated the trends in survival of 445 patients with pPCL diagnosed between 1973 and 2009 [31]. The median OS based on periods of diagnosis was 5, 6, 4, and 12 months for those diagnosed during 1973–1995, 1996–2000, 2001–2005, and 2006–2009, respectively. The improvement in OS seen between 2006 and 2009 was suspected to be due to the upfront incorporation of novel agent therapies [31]. However, early mortality was still 15 % within the first month during the recent period reflecting the aggressiveness of the disease [31]. Several recent single-institution series also report on the recent improvements in outcomes of patients with pPCL after treatment with novel agents (Table 1.1).

Treatment

There are no randomized clinical trials reporting outcomes exclusively in any of the PCL populations. Thus, most information on outcomes is obtained through retrospective, single-, or multi-institution experiences.

Table 1.1 Studies evaluating outcomes in patients with pPCL treated with novel agent therapy

Study (time period)	No. of patients	Induction regimens used	Outcomes
Katodritou et al. [48] (2000–2013)	25 pPCL	Bortezomib-based	ORR: 89 % OS: 18 months
D'Arena et al. (2006–2010)	29 pPCL	Bortezomib-based	ORR: 79 % OS: 55 % at 24-month follow-up
Musto et al. [49] (2002–2006)	12 (8 pPCL and 4 sPCL)	Bortezomib-based	pPCL: ORR: 92 % PFS and OS at 21 months: not reached
Musto et al. [50] (2009–2011)	23 pPCL	Lenalidomide–dexamethasone	ORR: 74 % OS: *ASCT used*: not reached *ASCT not used*: 12 months
Talamo et al. [51] (2006–2011)	17 (12 pPCL and 5 sPCL)	Novel agents—thalidomide, lenalidomide, bortezomib	ORR: 82 % OS: pPCL—21 months; sPCL—4 months
Usmani et al. [17] (1990–2006)	27 pPCL	TT1: conventional multi-agent chemotherapy TT2: thalidomide-based TT3: bortezomib-based	OS: 21.6 months (Only thalidomide and bortezomib-based regimens linked with improved OS)
Mahindra et al. [47] (1995–2006)	147 pPCL	Autologous-SCT (<30 % received novel agents) Allogeneic SCT (<30 % received novel agents)	Autologous-SCT 3-year OS: 64 % 3-year NRM: 5 % Allogeneic SCT 3-year OS: 39 % 3-year NRM: 41 %

(continued)

Table 1.1 (continued)

Study (time period)	No. of patients	Induction regimens used	Outcomes
Lebovic et al. [44] (2003–2009)	25 (13 pPCL; 12 sPCL)	Bortezomib or lenalidomide based	OS: 28.4 months
Pagano et al. [14] (2000–2008)	73 pPCL	Thalidomide/bortezomib-based (26 %) Chemotherapy (74 %)	ORR: 63 % in Thal/bortezomib group OS: 12.6 months for Thal and bortezomib-based regimens

Conventional Chemotherapy

The prognosis of pPCL and sPCL after conventional chemotherapy without novel agents prior to 2000 has been poor, and the median survival has typically remained under 12 months. There is limited improvement in response rates and survival gained from multi-agent conventional chemotherapy, such as vincristine, adri-amycin, and dexamethasone (VAD)-based regimens compared with traditional alkylator–steroid combination therapies such as melphalan and dexamethasone [8, 10].

Novel Agent Therapies

The introduction of immunomodulators and proteasome inhibitors has significantly improved survival of MM patients [32]. These agents also improve outcome of pPCL, but the benefit is less prominent [31]. There are limited number of prospective studies evaluating novel agents in pPCL, but several retrospective studies provide supportive information on their efficacy.

Immunomodulators

Thalidomide: Few studies have reported conflicting results in small numbers of PCL patients. One study reported on three pPCL patients that experienced two PRs and one SD for an average duration of 14 months with single-agent thalidomide while one patient with sPCL did not respond [33]. However, Pettrucci et al. [34] reported on five cases of pPCL and sPCL treated with single-agent thalidomide that did not show any response and all patients died within 120 days of treatment. Finally, thalidomide's decreased activity in extramedullary MM [35–37] makes its use in the routine treatment of patients presenting with pPCL less attractive. However, it can still be utilized in combination with other agents quite effectively in both patients with pPCL and sPCL.

Lenalidomide: The combination of lenalidomide with dexam-ethasone was evaluated in a phase 2 study of 23 newly diagnosed pPCL patients. Of these patients, 61 and 35 % achieved a PR and

VGPR [38]. The OS and PFS were 63 and 52 %, respectively, suggesting the efficacy of this combination in comparison with historical outcomes of patients with pPCL [38]. Furthermore, lenalidomide is also effective in the treatment of patients with relapsed pPCL [39, 40].

Pomalidomide: This is the latest immunomodulator drug available for the treatment of MM. Even though there are no reports of its activity specifically in pPCL or sPCL, pomalidomide plus low-dose dexamethasone resulted in two complete and two partial responses among 13 patients with extramedullary disease [41]. This is promising for activity in patients with pPCL who also tend to have extramedullary features.

Proteasome Inhibitors

The incorporation of bortezomib into the induction and salvage regimens of patients with MM has led to improvements in their survival. Similar improvements in the outcomes of pPCL and sPCL have also been reported in various single-institution studies. A large prospective analysis of 29 newly diagnosed pPCL patients treated with bortezomib-based regimens reported an overall response rate of 79 % of which 38 % were VGPRs [42]. The two-year PFS and OS were 40 and 55 %. In the Greek experience reported by Katodritou et al., bortezomib-based regimens were administered in 25 patients with pPCL and 17 with sPCL [43]. Objective response rates and OS were 69 % and 13 months, respectively [43]. Lebovic et al. reported on 13 patients with pPCL and 12 patients with sPCL. The bortezomib-treated patients had a median survival of 28 months compared with 4 months for the non-bortezomib-treated group $(P < 0.001)$ [44]. However, the pPCL patients who underwent treatment on the Total Therapy 3 protocol, which incorporates bortezomib, did not experience an improved survival compared with prior pPCL patients treated with the preceding Total Therapy regimens that lacked the use of bortezomib [17].

Autologous Stem Cell Transplant

High-dose chemotherapy followed by stem cell rescue or autologous stem cell transplant (ASCT) has been incorporated into the treatment paradigm of most patients with MM who are medically eligible [45]. Given the poor prognosis associated with pPCL, ASCT has been widely adopted as an integral part of therapy for patients with pPCL. The retrospective series from the Mayo Clinic demonstrated an improved median OS of 34 versus 11 months when comparing patients who received and did not received an ASCT [8]. A retrospective analysis performed by the European Group for Blood and Marrow Transplantation on 272 pPCL patients undergoing ASCT between 1980 and 2006 showed a higher treatment-related mortality (TRM) in the patients with pPCL compared with patients with MM [46]. The median PFS and median OS for patients with pPCL were 14.3 and 25.7 months, respectively [46]. The Center for International Blood and Marrow Transplant Research (CIBMTR) evaluated 97 pPCL patients who received an upfront ASCT between 1995 and 2006 [47]. The three-year PFS and OS were 34 and 64 %, respectively, with a trend toward superior OS in patients who received a tandem ASCT compared with those receiving a single ASCT [47]. The reported non-relapse mortality at three years was 5 %.

Allogeneic Stem Cell Transplant

The retrospective CIBMTR study also evaluated 50 patients who received an allogeneic SCT between 1995 and 2006 [47]. Most patients (68 %) received a myeloablative conditioning regimen, whereas the rest received a non-myeloablative or reduced intensity conditioning regimen. The cumulative incidence of relapse at 3 years was 38 %, but the TRM at 3 years was 41 % resulting in a 3-year OS of 39 % [47].

General Approach to the Treatment of PPCL and SPCL

We propose a risk-adapted approach when managing patients with plasma cell malignancies. Given the highly aggressive nature of pPCL, rapid cytoreduction of the disease is required in order to avoid early mortality. Thus, we recommend induction therapy with a combination of novel agent therapies such as both proteasome inhibitors and immunomodulators such as VRD (bortezomib, lenalidomide, and dexamethasone). In some patients with pPCL with an extensive burden of disease, more aggressive combination regimens such as VDT-PACE could be utilized. After induction therapy in transplant eligible pPCL patients, an upfront ASCT is recommended in order to achieve a deeper response and longer disease control. Given the higher likelihood of prolonged disease remission in patients undergoing allogeneic SCT compared with ASCT, the former can be considered in patients with an available fully matched sibling or unrelated donor. However, the higher risk of TRM with allogeneic SCTs should be taken into consideration and preferentially performed in the setting of a clinical trial. At a minimum, the patient's stem cells should at least be harvested and stored for use for an ASCT in the future if not performed in the upfront setting. Although the data are scarce, post-ASCT maintenance is highly recommended given the high propensity for early relapse. These maintenance regimens can include either bortezomib, lenalidomide, or both in combination-based regimens based on the significant disease control experienced by patients with MM including those with high-risk cytogenetics. Patients with pPCL not eligible for ASCT-based options should still be treated with combinations of novel agents as induction therapy with plans for indefinite maintenance therapy to keep the disease controlled.

For patients with sPCL, if medically fit, clinical trials utilizing novel agents should be considered; however, many trials exclude such patients from participation. Nevertheless, more intensive regimens such as VDT-PACE can also be considered, but this should be followed by a plan for consolidative therapy with either an ASCT or an allogeneic SCT. Whereas for transplant ineligible patients or previously transplanted patients, prolonged maintenance therapy must be continued.

Future Considerations

There is much improvement to be made in the management of patients with pPCL and sPCL especially in early detection and intervention. The correct diagnosis of pPCL and sPCL is dependent upon the ability of the hematopathologist to recognize circulating PCs on a peripheral blood smear. This expertise may vary among institutions making the diagnosis subjective, and hence, uniform techniques and criteria are needed to improve the ability to diagnose PCL uniformly. This will allow for the early detection or screening for PCL which could lead to the incorporation of earlier interventions and therefore change the natural history of the disease. Finally, clinical trials testing newer therapeutic agents in pPCL and sPCL patients should be conducted to allow for the continued improvement in survival outcomes.

References

1. Siegel RL, Miller KD, Jemal A. Cancer statistics, 2015. CA Cancer J Clin. 2015;65:5–29.
2. Gluzinski A, Reichenstein M. Myeloma and leucaemia lymphatica plasmocellularis. Wein Klin Wochenschr. 1906;336–339.
3. Kyle RA, Maldonado JE, Bayrd ED. Plasma cell leukemia. Report on 17 cases. Arch Intern Med. 1974;133:813–8.
4. Kyle RA, et al. Criteria for the classification of monoclonal gammopathies, multiple myeloma and related disorders: a report of the International Myeloma Working Group. Br J Haematol. 2003;121:749–57.
5. Albarracin F, Fonseca R. Plasma cell leukemia. Blood Rev. 2011;25:107–12.
6. Blade J, Kyle RA. Nonsecretory myeloma, immunoglobulin D myeloma, and plasma cell leukemia. Hematol Oncol Clin North Am. 1999;13:1259–72.
7. Sher T, Miller KC, Deeb G, Lee K, Chanan-Khan A. Plasma cell leukaemia and other aggressive plasma cell malignancies. Br J Haematol. 2010;150:418–27.
8. Tiedemann RE, Gonzalez-Paz N, Kyle RA, et al. Genetic aberrations and survival in plasma cell leukemia. Leukemia. 2008;22:1044–52.
9. Noel P, Kyle RA. Plasma cell leukemia: an evaluation of response to therapy. Am J Med. 1987;83:1062–8.
10. Dimopoulos MA, Palumbo A, Delasalle KB, Alexanian R. Primary plasma cell leukaemia. Br J Haematol. 1994;88:754–9.

11. Garcia-Sanz R, Orfao A, Gonzalez M, et al. Primary plasma cell leukemia: clinical, immunophenotypic, DNA ploidy, and cytogenetic characteristics. Blood. 1999;93:1032–7.
12. Colovic M, Jankovic G, Suvajdzic N, Milic N, Dordevic V, Jankovic S. Thirty patients with primary plasma cell leukemia: a single center experience. Med Oncol. 2008;25:154–60.
13. Peijing Q, Yan X, Yafei W, et al. A retrospective analysis of thirty-one cases of plasma cell leukemia from a single center in China. Acta Haematol. 2009;121:47–51.
14. Pagano L, Valentini CG, De Stefano V, et al. Primary plasma cell leukemia: a retrospective multicenter study of 73 patients. Ann Oncol. 2011;22:1628–35.
15. Fernandez de Larrea C, Kyle RA, Durie BG, et al. Plasma cell leukemia: consensus statement on diagnostic requirements, response criteria and treatment recommendations by the International Myeloma Working Group. Leukemia. 2013;27:780–91.
16. Yamamoto JF, Goodman MT. Patterns of leukemia incidence in the United States by subtype and demographic characteristics, 1997–2002. Cancer Causes Control: CCC. 2008;19:379–90.
17. Usmani SZ, Nair B, Qu P, et al. Primary plasma cell leukemia: clinical and laboratory presentation, gene-expression profiling and clinical outcome with total therapy protocols. Leukemia. 2012;26:2398–405.
18. Woodruff RK, Malpas JS, Paxton AM, Lister TA. Plasma cell leukemia (PCL): a report on 15 patients. Blood. 1978;52:839–45.
19. Perez-Andres M, Almeida J, Martin-Ayuso M, et al. Clonal plasma cells from monoclonal gammopathy of undetermined significance, multiple myeloma and plasma cell leukemia show different expression profiles of molecules involved in the interaction with the immunological bone marrow microenvironment. Leukemia. 2005;19:449–55.
20. Kraj M, Kopec-Szlezak J, Poglod R, Kruk B. Flow cytometric immunophenotypic characteristics of 36 cases of plasma cell leukemia. Leuk Res. 2011;35:169–76.
21. Buda G, Carulli G, Orciuolo E, et al. CD23 expression in plasma cell leukaemia. Br J Haematol. 2010;150:724–5.
22. Guikema JE, Hovenga S, Vellenga E, et al. CD27 is heterogeneously expressed in multiple myeloma: low CD27 expression in patients with high-risk disease. Br J Haematol. 2003;121:36–43.
23. Avet-Loiseau H, Daviet A, Brigaudeau C, et al. Cytogenetic, interphase, and multicolor fluorescence in situ hybridization analyses in primary plasma cell leukemia: a study of 40 patients at diagnosis, on behalf of the Intergroupe Francophone du Myelome and the Groupe Francais de Cytogenetique Hematologique. Blood. 2001;97:822–5.
24. Fonseca R, Blood E, Rue M, et al. Clinical and biologic implications of recurrent genomic aberrations in myeloma. Blood. 2003;101:4569–75.
25. Avet-Loiseau H, Roussel M, Campion L, et al. Cytogenetic and therapeutic characterization of primary plasma cell leukemia: the IFM experience. Leukemia. 2012;26:158–9.

26. Chiecchio L, Dagrada GP, White HE, et al. Frequent upregulation of MYC in plasma cell leukemia. Genes Chromosom Cancer. 2009;48:624–36.

27. Bezieau S, Devilder MC, Avet-Loiseau H, et al. High incidence of N and K-Ras activating mutations in multiple myeloma and primary plasma cell leukemia at diagnosis. Hum Mutat. 2001;18:212–24.

28. Corradini P, Ladetto M, Voena C, et al. Mutational activation of N- and K-ras oncogenes in plasma cell dyscrasias. Blood. 1993;81:2708–13.

29. Chang H, Qi XY, Claudio J, Zhuang L, Patterson B, Stewart AK. Analysis of PTEN deletions and mutations in multiple myeloma. Leuk Res. 2006;30:262–5.

30. Egan JB, Shi CX, Tembe W, et al. Whole-genome sequencing of multiple myeloma from diagnosis to plasma cell leukemia reveals genomic initiating events, evolution, and clonal tides. Blood. 2012;120:1060–6.

31. Gonsalves WI, Rajkumar SV, Go RS, et al. Trends in survival of patients with primary plasma cell leukemia: a population-based analysis. Blood. 2014;124:907–12.

32. Kumar SK, Rajkumar SV, Dispenzieri A, et al. Improved survival in multiple myeloma and the impact of novel therapies. Blood. 2008;111:2516–20.

33. Johnston RE, Abdalla SH. Thalidomide in low doses is effective for the treatment of resistant or relapsed multiple myeloma and for plasma cell leukaemia. Leuk Lymphoma. 2002;43:351–4.

34. Petrucci MT, Martini V, Levi A, et al. Thalidomide does not modify the prognosis of plasma cell leukemia patients: experience of a single center. Leuk Lymphoma. 2007;48:180–2.

35. Katodritou E, Gastari V, Verrou E, et al. Extramedullary (EMP) relapse in unusual locations in multiple myeloma: is there an association with precedent thalidomide administration and a correlation of special biological features with treatment and outcome? Leuk Res. 2009;33:1137–40.

36. Candoni A, Simeone E, Fanin R. Extramedullary progression of multiple myeloma under thalidomide therapy despite concomitant response of medullary disease. Am J Hematol. 2008;83:680–1.

37. Rosinol L, Cibeira MT, Blade J, et al. Extramedullary multiple myeloma escapes the effect of thalidomide. Haematologica. 2004;89:832–6.

38. Musto P, Simeon V, Martorelli MC, et al. Lenalidomide and low-dose dexamethasone for newly diagnosed primary plasma cell leukemia. Leukemia. 2014;28:222–5.

39. Musto P, Pietrantuono G, Guariglia R, et al. Salvage therapy with lenalidomide and dexamethasone in relapsed primary plasma cell leukemia. Leuk Res. 2008;32:1637–8.

40. Guglielmelli T, Merlini R, Giugliano E, Saglio G. Lenalidomide, melphalan, and prednisone association is an effective salvage therapy in relapsed plasma cell leukaemia. J Oncol. 2009;2009:867380.

41. Short KD, Rajkumar SV, Larson D, et al. Incidence of extramedullary disease in patients with multiple myeloma in the era of novel therapy, and the activity of pomalidomide on extramedullary myeloma. Leukemia. 2011;25:906–8.

42. D'Arena G, Valentini CG, Pietrantuono G, et al. Frontline chemotherapy with bortezomib-containing combinations improves response rate and survival in primary plasma cell leukemia: a retrospective study from GIMEMA Multiple Myeloma Working Party. Ann Oncol. 2012;23:1499–502.
43. Katodritou E, Terpos E, Kelaidi C, et al. Treatment with bortezomib-based regimens improves overall response and predicts for survival in patients with primary or secondary plasma cell leukemia: analysis of the Greek myeloma study group. Am J Hematol. 2014;89:145–50.
44. Lebovic D, Zhang L, Alsina M, et al. Clinical outcomes of patients with plasma cell leukemia in the era of novel therapies and hematopoietic stem cell transplantation strategies: a single-institution experience. Clin Lymphoma Myeloma Leuk. 2011;11:507–11.
45. Mikhael JR, Dingli D, Roy V, et al. Management of newly diagnosed symptomatic multiple myeloma: updated Mayo stratification of myeloma and risk-adapted therapy (mSMART) consensus guidelines 2013. Mayo Clin Proc. 2013;88:360–76.
46. Drake MB, Iacobelli S, van Biezen A, et al. Primary plasma cell leukemia and autologous stem cell transplantation. Haematologica. 2010;95:804–9.
47. Mahindra A, Kalaycio ME, Vela-Ojeda J, et al. Hematopoietic cell transplantation for primary plasma cell leukemia: results from the Center for International Blood and Marrow Transplant Research. Leukemia. 2012;26:1091–7.
48. Katodritou E, Terpos E, Kelaidi C, et al. Treatment with bortezomib-based regimens improves overall response and predicts for survival in patients with primary or secondary plasma cell leukemia: analysis of the Greek myeloma study group. Am J Hematol. 2013.
49. Musto P, Rossini F, Gay F, et al. Efficacy and safety of bortezomib in patients with plasma cell leukemia. Cancer. 2007;109:2285–90.
50. Musto P, Simeon V, Martorelli MC, et al. Lenalidomide and low-dose dexamethasone for newly diagnosed primary plasma cell leukemia. Leukemia. 2013.
51. Talamo G, Dolloff NG, Sharma K, Zhu J, Malysz J. Clinical features and outcomes of plasma cell leukemia: a single-institution experience in the era of novel agents. Rare Tumors. 2012;4:e39.

Chapter 2
Plasmacytoma—Current Approach to Diagnosis and Management

Nidhi Tandon, MD and Shaji K. Kumar, MD

Introduction

Plasma cell dyscrasias (PCD) are characterized by an abnormal accumulation of monoclonal plasma cells typically producing high levels of monoclonal immunoglobulins or paraproteins. The spectrum of PCD ranges from monoclonal gammopathy of undetermined significance (MGUS) to symptomatic multiple myeloma (MM). The American Cancer Society has estimated 26,850 new myeloma cases in the USA in 2015 with an estimated 11,240 deaths [1].

A minority of patients with plasma cell malignancies present with either a single bone lesion, or less commonly, a soft tissue mass made up of monoclonal plasma cells. The solitary plasma-

N. Tandon, MD
Division of Hematology, Mayo Clinic, 200 First Street SW, Rochester, MN 55902, USA
e-mail: tandon.nidhi@mayo.edu

S.K. Kumar, MD (✉)
Division of Hematology, Department of Medicine, Mayo Clinic, 200 First Street SW, Rochester, MN 55902, USA
e-mail: kumar.shaji@mayo.edu

© Springer Science+Business Media New York 2017
T.M. Zimmerman and S.K. Kumar (eds.),
Biology and Management of Unusual Plasma Cell Dyscrasias,
DOI 10.1007/978-1-4419-6848-7_2

cytoma (SP) is characterized by a localized accumulation of neo-plastic monoclonal plasma cells in the absence of other features of systemic plasma cell proliferative disorder (i.e., anemia, hyper-calcemia, renal insufficiency, or multiple lytic bone lesions) [2–4].

SP can be classified into 2 groups depending upon its location; solitary plasmacytoma of the bone (SBP), if the tumor involves an osseous site and extramedullary plasmacytoma (EMP), if it involves an extra osseous site [2]. SBP mostly occurs in the bones of the axial skeleton, such as vertebra and skull [2, 5]. EMP is most often located in the head and neck region, mainly in the upper aero digestive tract such as the nasal cavity and nasopharynx, but may also occur in the gastrointestinal tract, urinary bladder, central nervous system, thyroid, breast, testes, parotid gland, lymph nodes, and skin [6–8].

The reason as to why some patients develop MM and others develop SP is not well understood, but it may be related to dif-ferences in cellular adhesion molecules or chemokine receptor expression profiles of the malignant plasma cells [9]. The diagnosis and management of patients with SP require the same range of clinical and laboratory expertise as for patients with MM, and a close liaison among the hematologist, radiotherapist, and surgeon is crucial for planning optimum care of these patients [10].

Epidemiology

SP is a rare form of plasma cell neoplasm and represents 3–5 % of all PCD according to the published literature [2]. An analysis of the surveillance, epidemiology, and end results (SEER) database from 1992 to 2004 demonstrated that the incidence of MM ($n = 23,544$; IR 5.35/100,000 person years) is 16 times higher than SP overall ($n = 1543$; IR = 0.34), and incidence of SBP was 40 % higher than EMP ($p < 0.0001$) [11].

The median age of the patients with either SBP or EMP is 55 years, which is much lower than the median age of 67–71 years for patients with MM. The incidence rate rises exponentially with advancing age; however, it is less prominent in older age group as compared to MM. The male to female ratio is 2:1. The incidence is highest in Blacks and lowest in Asians and Pacific Islanders [11–13].

Clinical Features

The clinical presentation is defined by the location and size of the plasmacytoma. The most common presenting symptom is pain due to bony destruction. Patients with vertebral involvement may also have evidence of spinal cord or nerve root compression [13–15]. Involvement of the base of the skull can present with cranial nerve palsies [16, 17].

SBP most commonly affects bones involved with active hematopoiesis; hence, the axial skeleton is more commonly involved than the appendicular skeleton, particularly the vertebra [13–15]. The thoracic vertebrae are more commonly involved than the lumbar, sacral, or cervical spine [4]. Around 20 % of patients with SBP have affection of ribs, sternum, clavicle, or scapula [18].

Most patients with EMP present with symptoms related to the location of the soft tissue mass. Approximately 80 % of the EMP involve mucosa associated lymphoid tissue of the upper respiratory tract; 75 % of which involve the oro-nasopharynx and paranasal sinuses producing rhinorrhea, epistaxis, or nasal obstruction [7, 19]. Other less commonly involved sites are the gastrointestinal tract [20], lung [21, 22], pleura [23], liver [24], bladder [25], testes [26], ovary [27], skin [28], lymph nodes [29], and central nervous system [30].

Localized amyloidosis can be a feature of both SBP and EMP [31, 32]. By definition, evidence of end-organ damage attributable to PCD like anemia (i.e., hemoglobin <10 g/dL or 2 g/dL below normal), hypercalcemia (i.e., serum calcium >11 mg/dL or 1 mg/dL higher than the upper limit of normal), or renal insufficiency (i.e., serum creatinine >2 mg/dL or creatinine clearance <40 mL/min) is not present in SP [33].

Diagnosis

The evaluation of a patient with suspected SP requires the following [34, 35]:

1. Biopsy of the single lytic bone lesion or soft tissue mass.

2. Complete blood count (CBC) with peripheral smear examination.
3. Biochemical screen including serum creatinine, calcium, albumin, lactate dehydrogenase, beta-2 microglobulin, and C-reactive protein.
4. Serum protein electrophoresis (SPEP) with immunofixation (IF) and quantitation of immunoglobulins, and a serum free light-chain (SFLC) assay.
5. 24-hour urine collection for total protein, electrophoresis (UPEP) with immunofixation (IF).
6. Unilateral bone marrow aspiration and biopsy.
7. Skeletal survey and either a positron emission tomography/computed tomography (PET/CT) scan or a magnetic resonance imaging (MRI) of the entire spine and pelvis.

The diagnostic criteria for SP require the following [33]:

1. Histopathological confirmation of a monoclonal plasma cell infiltration of a single lytic bone lesion or soft tissue mass.
2. Absence of clonal plasma cells on a random bone marrow sample.
3. No additional lesions on bone survey or MRI of the spine and pelvis.
4. Absence of end-organ damage such as CRAB lesions (increased calcium, renal insufficiency, anemia, or multiple osteolytic bone lesions on skeletal survey, CT scan, or PET–CT scan) that can be attributed to plasma cell proliferative disorder.

A biopsy of the suspected lesion can usually be obtained using computed tomography (CT) or MRI guidance. Fine needle aspiration cytology is inadequate for diagnosis [34]. Monoclonality and/or an aberrant plasma cell phenotype should be demonstrated with useful markers being CD19, CD56, CD27, CD117, and cyclin D1 [36].

The presence of monoclonal protein (M protein) in the serum or urine of patients with SP has been noted in 24–72 % of patients in various series [2, 5, 13, 37, 38]. The level of the M protein is usually low (usually <1 g/dL) and may or may not disappear with treatment. The presence of M protein is much more common in SBP than EMP [2, 8, 13]. A cohort of 116 patients with SBP were evaluated to develop a risk stratification model for progression to

MM and 47 % ($n = 54$) of the patients were found to have an abnormal FLC ratio [39]. In another series of 43 patients, 48 % of patients were found to have an abnormal involved SFLC value, and 64 % had an abnormal SFLC ratio at diagnosis [40].

Flow cytometry studies and molecular detection of heavy- and light-chain gene rearrangements may reveal clonal plasma cells in the bone marrow of some patients who have no evidence of infiltration on light microscopy. Some patients with SP may demonstrate up to 10 % clonal plasma cells on the bone marrow and are considered as having both SP and MGUS. These patients are treated in a similar fashion to SP, but have a higher risk of progression to symptomatic myeloma [35].

Like MM, SBP has a lytic appearance on plain radiographs. In most patients, the lesion is purely lytic and has a clear margin and a narrow zone of transition to normal surrounding bone. CT and particularly MRI depict the extent of lesion more clearly than an X-ray. The MRI appearance of SBP is consistent with that of a focal area of bone marrow replacement; the signal intensity is similar to muscle on T1-weighted images and hyperintense relative to muscle on T2-weighted images [2]. MRI is a useful tool to identify soft tissue disease and "breakout" lesions in which a focal area of disease breaks through the cortex of bone into the soft tissues (including epidural spread) [41]. Also, MRI is important for delineating the extra osseous soft tissue component in the vertebrae, which may impinge on the spinal cord or spinal nerve roots [42]. The role of MRI of the thoracic and lumbosacral spine to seek additional foci of marrow involvement in patients with an apparent SBP was prospectively evaluated by Moulopoulos et al. MRI showed additional abnormalities in 4 out of 12 patients, with signal characteristics identical to those of the primary tumor. In all 4 patients, the abnormal protein persisted at greater than 50 % of the pretreatment value following definitive RT. In contrast, the M protein disappeared or was reduced by greater than 50 % in 5 of the 6 patients with secretory disease and without additional marrow abnormalities. One of the 4 patients progressed to MM 10 months after diagnosis with new lesions on conventional radiographs in the same areas as detected previously by MRI [43]. Also, Liebross et al. [44] reported that among 23 patients with thoracolumbar SBP, 7 of 8 patients who had SBP on plain radiographs alone developed MM as compared to only 1 of 7 patients who also had negative results on MRI of the spine. Thus, whole-body MRI or spine and pelvic MRI (if WB-MRI is not available) should be part of the staging procedures in patients with SP to better assess the extent of the local tumor and reveal occult lesions elsewhere [42].

Focal lesions on FDG–PET or PET/CT scan are defined as well-circumscribed areas of increased uptake relative to the marrow background that are thought to represent areas of tumor involvement, measuring at least 5 mm in one dimension. Areas of focal uptake on FDG–PET images resolve very quickly with effective treatment, similar to the time course of M protein normalization in secretory disease [41]. The sensitivity of FDG–PET in detecting myelomatous involvement is approximately 85–96 %, and its specificity is approximately 77–90 % in different studies [45, 46]. Schirrmeister et al. [47] assessed the accuracy of PET scan in patients with presumed SP. Additional lesions, not identified by standard staging methods, were found in 4 of the 11 patients with SBP altering therapy.

It has been estimated that one-third of patients with an apparently SPB by bone survey have evidence of other plasma cell tumors on PET/CT or MRI of the spine; these patients are at greater risk for progression to multiple myeloma [48–50]. The relative advantages of MRI compared to FDG–PET and integrated PET/CT are its more widespread availability and superior spatial and contrast resolution, particularly for involvement of skull, skull base, and face. The relative disadvantages of MRI compared to FDG–PET are the time and expense required for a thorough examination of the skeletal system, its limited field of view to the region under examination, and its contraindicated use in some patients (such as patients with pacemakers, cochlear implants, and aneurysm clips). Also, the focal lesions seen on MRI will take, typically, months to years to resolve, and hence, although MRI is ideal to document "completeness" of response, FDG–PET or integrated PET/CT is more useful for monitoring short-term response [41].

Zamagni et al. prospectively compared 18F-FDG PET–CT, MRI of the spine–pelvis and skeletal survey for baseline assessment of bone disease in a series of 46 patients with newly diagnosed MM. Overall, PET–CT was superior to X-rays in 46 % of patients, including 19 % with negative skeletal survey. PET–CT scans of the spine and pelvis failed to show abnormal findings in 30 % of the patients with lesions on MRI. In contrast, in 35 % of patients PET–CT enabled the detection of lesions which were out of the field of view of MRI [51]. A prospective trial compared MRI and PET/CT for appraisal of plasmacytoma and demonstrated an equivalent or higher sensitivity, specificity, positive predictive value, and negative predictive value for baseline staging of plasmacytomas with PET/CT as compared to MRI. However, this study was limited by small sample size ($n = 23$) [52].

Treatment

The standard of care for SP is radiotherapy (RT) given with curative intent. Surgery may be required for patients with retropulsed bone, structural instability of the bone, or rapidly progressive neurological symptoms from spinal cord compression. If a complete surgical resection was performed as part of the diagnosis, the role of adjuvant RT is not well defined [37].

A variety of treatment strategies have been tried in SBP and EMP as summarized in Tables 2.1 and 2.2.

Radiation

Definitive local radiotherapy (RT) is the treatment of choice for SP. The evidence comes largely from retrospective studies of small numbers of patients due to rarity of the disease. In a review of 206 patients with SBP, local relapse occurred in 21(14 %) out of 148 patients who received RT alone compared with 4(80 %) out of 5 patients who were treated with surgery with or without chemotherapy. Surgery (RT versus partial or complete resection and RT) did not influence the 10-year probability of local control [56]. The largest retrospective study included 258 patients with SBP ($n = 206$) or EMP ($n = 52$). The treatments included RT alone ($n = 214$), RT plus chemotherapy ($n = 34$), and surgery alone ($n = 8$). Five-year rates of overall survival (OS), disease-free survival (DFS), and local control (LC) were 74, 50, and 86 %, respectively. The median time to MM development was 21 months (range 2–135), with a 5-year probability of 45 %. Patients who

Table 2.1 Representative treatment results from major studies in solitary bone plasmacytoma (SBP) from the literature

Author, year	n	Therapy given	F/U	10 year LC (%)	10 year PMM (%)	10 year OS (%)
Bataille et al. [15], 1981	114	95—surgery + RT Rest—surgery/ Surgery + CT/ Unknown/no Rx	Few weeks to 24 years	88	58	68.5
Chak et al. [53], 1987	65	RT/surgery + RT/chemo	87 month	95	77	52
Frassica et al. [13], 1989	46	43—RT (median = 39.75 Gy) 3—surgery	90 month	89	54	45
Liebross et al. [43], 1998	57	RT (median = 50 Gy)	–	96	51	11 year (median OS)
Tsang et al. [54], 2001	32	Majority—RT (median = 35 Gy) Others— surgery + RT/RT + chemo/IFN	95 month	78 (At 8 year)	64 (At 8 year)	65 (At 8 year)
Wilder et al. [55], 2002	60	RT (median = 46 Gy)	7.8 year	90	62	59
Knobel et al. [56], 2006	206	169—RT 32—RT + chemo 5—surgery	54 month	79	51	50

(continued)

Table 2.1 (continued)

Author, year	n	Therapy given	F/U	10 year LC (%)	10 year PMM (%)	10 year OS (%)
Ozahin et al. [57], 2006	206	Majority—RT Others— RT + chemo/surgery/chemo	56 month	79	72	52
Kilciksiz et al. [58], 2008	57	30—RT 26—RT + surgery 1—unknown	2.4 year	94	4.1 year (median myeloma-free survival)	68

Table 2.2 Representative treatment results from major studies in solitary extramedullary plasmacytoma (EMP) from the literature

Author, year	n	Therapy given	F/U	10 year LC (%)	10 year PMM (%)	10 year OS (%)
Knowling et al. [59], 1983	25	22—RT (35–40 Gy) 3—surgery	71 month	88	28	43
Soeson et al. [60], 1991	25	RT/surgery/surgery + RT or chemo/chemo	44 month	88	–	50
Liebross et al. [61], 1999	22	18—RT (median = 50 Gy) 2—surgery 2—surgery + RT	–	95	32	56
Tsang et al. [54], 2001	14	Majority—RT (median = 35 Gy) Others— Surgery + RT/RT + chemo/IFN	95 month	93 (At 8 year)	16 (At 8 year)	65 (At 8 year)
Strojan et al. [62], 2002	26	12—RT 15—surgery + RT 4—surgery	61 month	87	8	61
Chao et al. [63], 2005	16	RT (median = 45 Gy)	66 month	100	31	54
Ozahin et al. [57], 2006	52	Majority—RT Others— RT + chemo/surgery/chemo	56 month	74	36	72
Kilciksiz et al. [58], 2008	23	10—RT 12—RT + surgery 1—unknown	2.4 year	95	7.4 year	89

received localized RT had a lower rate of local relapse (12 %) than those who did not (60 %). Younger age and tumor size <4 cm were favorable for OS; and younger age, extramedullary localization, and RT were favorable for DFS on multivariate analysis [57].

The optimal dose of radiation for SP has not been established. Tsang et al. demonstrated that the radiation was not associated with local failure (8-year local DFS was 100 % for 30 Gy, 81 % for 35 Gy, and 80 % for 40 Gy, $p = 0.50$), or progression to myeloma in patients with SP. The tumor bulk (size > 5 cm) was found to be the most significant factor negatively influencing local control [54]. Mendenhall et al. [64] observed a 6 % incidence of local failure with doses of at least 40 Gy which was superior to 31 % incidence of local failure with lower doses among 81 patients with SP. Knobel et al. [56] evaluated 206 patients with SBP out of which 148 patients received RT with a median dose of 40 Gy and found no dose–response relationship was observed for doses higher than 30 Gy regardless of tumor size. Tournier-Rangeard et al. reviewed 17 patients with EMP and depicted that the 5-year LC was 90 % for patients who received ≥40 Gy compared with 40 % for those who received <40 Gy ($p = 0.031$). Patients who received ≥45 Gy had 100 % local disease control, but there was no statistical difference for LC from those who received a dose ≥40 Gy ($p = 0.39$). Five-year OS for patients who received ≥45 Gy or <45 Gy were 87.5 and 37.5 %, respectively ($p = 0.056$) [65]. In light of all these studies, strict dosing guidelines are difficult to recommend [56]. National comprehensive cancer network (NCCN) recommends >30 Gy to the involved field for SBP while >30 Gy to the involved field followed by surgery if necessary for the EMP [57]. The United Kingdom Myeloma Forum (UKMF) [37] recommends RT of at least 40 Gy in 20 fractions for both SBP and EMP routinely with a higher dose (up to 50 Gy in 25 fractions) for bulkier disease (>5 cm).

The clinical target volume should be designed to encompass all disease shown by CT or MRI scanning with a margin of at least 2 cm. For small bones, such as vertebrae, this will include the entire bone involved, together with one uninvolved vertebra above and below. For larger bones, the clinical target volume will not necessarily include the entire bone, as this would involve unnecessary irradiation of normal tissues [37]. Prophylactic regional lymph node irradiation is not necessary in SBP, whereas its addition to RT treatment portals in EMP provides excellent local control rates. However, in view of increased acute and late morbidity (especially xerostomia, which may not fully recover), it is not recommended routinely except for first echelon cervical lymph nodes in case of the primary sites involving Waldeyer's ring [37]. Conformal RT using parallel opposed fields is the most commonly used method to cover the PTV. However, IMRT technique might be considered in some cases to spare the critical structures, such as eyes and salivary glands [66].

After adequate radiotherapy, virtually all patients have relief of symptoms [2]. Patients not responding clinically to radiotherapy do not necessarily have residual tumor. They may have persistent symptoms and/or radiological changes as a result of existing bone destruction, and a repeat biopsy is advisable to clarify the situation in this circumstance [37].

The residual abnormalities on imaging post-treatment are invariable, difficult to assess, and do not correlate with outcome. Up to 50 % of patients show sclerosis and remineralization in up to 50 % of patients on plain radiography assessments [43]. The abnormalities of bone marrow and accompanying soft tissue mass may persist on MRI images, even after successful treatment [43]. Local control, defined as long-term clinical and radiographic stability, has been achieved in at least 90 % of cases [13, 43, 59].

Serial measurements of the monoclonal protein for at least 6 months after treatment are required to confirm disease radiosensitivity [2]. In most patients, the monoclonal protein is reduced markedly after completion of local RT. However, the rate of decline can be slow lasting several years [67]. The monoclonal protein disappears in about 20–50 % of patients, suggesting that all diseases were included within the RT field. The likelihood of disappearance of monoclonal protein is higher in patients in whom the pretreatment value is low. In many patients, the monoclonal protein persists despite adequate RT, indicating the presence of tumor beyond RT field. The condition of these patients may remain stable for a long time, and further treatment should be deferred until there is clear progression of the plasma cell disorder [2].

Surgery

Although most patients with SP can be treated with RT alone, surgical intervention may be necessary in some patients in whom the diagnosis of SP has not yet been made and they either present with or have rapid development of neurological dysfunction that requires laminectomy before radiotherapy [2]. An anterior approach usually allows the best access to the pathology, although some groups advocate a posterior approach to avoid the potential complications which can occur in trans-cavity access [68, 69]. Surgical procedures may also be required for patients with vertebral instability or a pathologic fracture of a long bone [2]. Loss of structural integrity requires some form of stabilization procedure, most frequently being posterior pedicle screw instrumentation. Vertebroplasty is likely to be of limited value in vertebral collapse due to SP because the degree of vertebral destruction renders the technique unsuitable [37].

Combined therapy is suggested when complete surgical tumor resection cannot be applied, and/or lymph node areas are affected. Alexiou et al. [7] reviewed more than 400 publications of EMP between 1905 and 1997 and reported that the median OS and DFS were better for surgery and RT compared with surgery alone for EMP involving the upper aero digestive (UAD) tract ($p = 0.0027$), but the difference was not statistically significant for non UAD EMP ($p = 0.62$). It is recommended that if surgery is required immediately or in the near future, it should be carried out before RT is commenced [37]. Surgery is more difficult in patients who have received RT. However, it is important to note that initial surgery may sometimes compromise RT, e.g., by the placing of metal supports, which may potentially shield areas of disease from effective radiation dose [69].

Adjuvant Chemotherapy

The role of adjuvant chemotherapy in SP has not been clearly defined at present. Although some studies have found that adjuvant therapy may prevent or delay progression to MM, most of the studies have reported no benefit with the early administration of chemotherapy [2, 5, 37]. More recently, even myeloablative therapy with stem cell support has been evaluated in high-risk patients with solitary bone plasmacytoma, but results are too premature to draw any conclusions given the long natural history of this disease [70].

Aviles et al. suggested benefit of 3 years of adjuvant melphalan and prednisolone after RT in OS and time to development of MM. Though this was a randomized-controlled trial, the number of patients ($n = 28$) was small to make any conclusion [71]. Holland et al. showed that the addition of chemotherapy delays the time for progression of SP to MM. However, its use was not associated with any decrease in rate of conversion to MM. Also, after progression to MM, the patients, who received chemotherapy, had the same OS as those who did not [72]. Furthermore, it is suggested that early exposure to chemotherapy may predispose to the development of resistant subclones and, therefore, limit later therapeutic options [2]. Besides in a series, 4 out of 7 patients with SBP who received adjuvant melphalan after RT developed secondary leukemia [73].

Therefore, given the lack of consistent data proving benefit from chemotherapy, currently there is no current role for adjuvant chemotherapy in the initial treatment of SP [37]. For the patients with tumors larger than 5 cm and high-grade histology and for tumors that have not responded to RT, adjuvant chemotherapy may be considered. Treatment schedules effective against multiple myeloma shall be utilized [38].

Adjuvant Bisphosphonates

Till date, there have been no reports about the role of bisphosphonates in preventing progression of SP to symptomatic multiple myeloma in the published literature. Bisphosphonates are not recommended for patients with SP, except in the setting of osteoporosis or osteopenia on bone mineral density studies, at doses used for osteoporosis [37, 74].

Follow-up

Serial and frequent measurement of M protein is required to judge disease response and progression to MM during surveillance. CBC, serum chemistry including creatinine and corrected calcium, SPEP with IF, serum FLCA, and 24 h urine for total protein, UPEP with IF should be repeated at 6-week intervals for the first 6 months and then with prolongation of clinic visits [66]. Bone survey is recommended annually or as clinically indicated. Bone marrow aspirate and biopsy and imaging studies including CT, MRI, or PET–CT may be done as clinically required [75].

Natural History and Prognosis

The median overall survival for SP is 7.5–12 years [2, 76]. The most common pattern of progression among patients with SP consists of new bone lesions, rising myeloma protein level, and development of marrow plasmacytosis [2]. There are three patterns of failure in these patients: local recurrence, development of new bone lesions (without MM), and progression to MM [77].

SBPs have a poorer prognosis in comparison with EMPs [37, 54, 58, 78]. SBP has a higher risk for progression to MM at a rate of 65–84 % in 10 years and 65–100 % in 15 years. Even after curative therapy, the median time to progression to MM is 2–3 years [13, 43, 56, 58, 72]. About 50–60 % of patients with EMP develop MM [38, 61, 79]. The OS at 10 years is 40–50 % for SBP as compared to 70 % for EMP [2, 8, 13]. Patients with EMP that progressed to MM had a 100 % 5-year survival rate as compared to 33 % for SBP [64]. When MM evolves, most patients have features of low tumor mass disease, a high rate of response to chemotherapy, and a prolonged survival [2].

A variety of factors have been found to influence the risk and frequency of progression from SP to MM. Age and tumor size at diagnosis are important prognostic factors. Bataille et al. depicted that older mean age and spinal involvement were more commonly associated with progression to MM in his review of 114 cases of SP [15]. Tsang et al. [54] reported that age more than 63 years and bulky tumors (>5 cm) had a much lower local control rate. A Turkish study concluded that age more than 55 years is unfavorable for myeloma-free survival in patients with SP [58]. However, the dimension of tumor at diagnosis is related to DFS and myeloma-free survival only on univariate analysis and not on multivariate analysis [58].

Histopathological factors play a key role in biology and hence the prognostication of SP. Anaplastic type plasmacytomas represents a higher histologic grade and a worse prognosis [80]. Kumar et al. studied angiogenesis in plasmacytoma and bone marrow biopsy samples from 25 patients with SP. High-grade angiogenesis was present in 64 % of plasmacytomas biopsy samples and none in bone marrow biopsy samples. Patients with high-grade angiogenesis in the plasmacytoma sample were more likely to progress to myeloma and had a shorter progression-free survival compared with patients with low-grade angiogenesis ($P = 0.02$) [81].

Reed et al. retrospectively reviewed 84 patients with SP (70 % —SBP and 30 %—EMP) who were treated with definitive RT during 1988 to 2008 and found that patients who had serum paraprotein detected at diagnosis had higher risk of progression to MM than those who did not (60 % vs. 39 %; $P = 0.016$) [82]. Low levels of uninvolved immunoglobulin may represent occult MM, and immunoparesis at presentation is found to be an adverse prognostic factor for the development of MM [83]. An abnormal FLC ratio is also independently associated with a higher risk of progression to myeloma. The risk of progression to MM at 5 years was 44 % in patients with an abnormal serum FLC ratio at diagnosis compared with 26 % in those with a normal FLC ratio in a study of patients with SBP [39].

The correlation between persistence of myeloma protein after RT and the development of MM has been demonstrated in several studies [15, 39, 84]. Dingli et al. constructed a risk stratification model using abnormal SFLC ratio at diagnosis and the level of M protein level at 1–2 years following diagnosis to identify patients with SBP at risk of progression to MM. Patients with a normal FLC ratio and M protein level less than 5 g/L (0.5 g/dL) were considered low risk; with either risk factor abnormal, intermediate risk; and with both an abnormal FLC ratio and M protein level of 5 g/L were considered high risk. The corresponding rates of progression at 5 years were significantly different in the low, intermediate, and high groups: 13, 26, and 62 %, respectively ($p < .001$) [39].

A multivariate analysis of prognostic factors in 60 patients with SBP at MD Anderson Cancer Centre concluded that persistence of M protein for more than 1 year after RT is the only independent adverse prognostic factor for myeloma-free and cause-specific survival. At a median follow-up of 7.8 years, only 1 of 13 patients with resolution of the paraprotein progressed to MM while over 90 % of patients with persistent paraprotein had progressed. Age, tumor size, and level of paraprotein at diagnosis had no independent prognostic value [55].

Multiple Solitary Plasmacytoma (±Recurrent)

Multiple solitary plasmacytomas, which may be recurrent, occur in up to 5 % of patients with an apparently solitary plasmacytoma. These may involve bone or soft tissue and occur concurrently or sequentially in the absence of bone marrow evidence of MM [34].

The treatment approaches to patients with multiple solitary plasmacytomas (±recurrent) are variable and are influenced by factors such as patient age, sites of recurrence, numbers of lesions, and disease-free interval. When 2 lesions occur concurrently at sites where RT fields will be limited and non-overlapping or isolated lesions develop at long intervals (i.e., >2 years), RT alone may be administered. Patients with more extensive disease or early relapse may benefit from systemic therapy ± autologous stem cell transplantation, as indicated for MM, with small cases series suggesting long-term disease control [34, 85, 86].

References

1. Siegel RL, Miller KD, Jemal A. Cancer statistics, 2015. CA Cancer J Clin. 2015;65(1):5–29.
2. Dimopoulos MA, Moulopoulos LA, Maniatis A, Alexanian R. Solitary plasmacytoma of bone and asymptomatic multiple myeloma. Blood. 2000;96:2037.

3. Jaffe ES, Harris NL, Stein H, Vardiman JW, editors. World Health Organization classification of tumours. Pathology and genetics of tumours of haematopoietic and lymphoid tissues. Lyon: IARC Press; 2001.

4. Swerdlow SH, Campo E, Harris NL, et al., editors. World Health Organization classification of tumours of haematopoietic and lymphoid tissues. Lyon: IARC Press; 2008.

5. Dimopoulos MA, Hamilos G. Solitary bone plasmacytoma and extramedullary plasmacytoma. Curr Treat Options Oncol. 2002;3 (3):255–9.

6. Wiltshaw E. The natural history of extramedullary plasmacytoma and its relation to solitary myeloma of bone and myelomatosis. Medicine. 1976;55 (3):217–38.

7. Alexiou C, Kau RJ, Dietzfelbinger H, et al. Extramedullary plasmacytoma: tumor occurrence and therapeutic concepts. Cancer. 1999;85(11):2305–14.

8. Galieni P, Cavo M, Pulsoni A, et al. Clinical outcome of extramedullary plasmacytoma. Haematologica. 2000;85(1):47–51.

9. Hughes M, Doig A, Soutar R. Solitary plasmacytoma and multiple myeloma: adhesion molecule and chemokine receptor expression patterns. Br J Haematol. 2007;137:486.

10. Guidelines on the diagnosis and management of multiple myeloma. Br J Haematol. 2001;115, 522–540.

11. Dores GM, Landgren O, McGlynn KA, Curtis RE, Linet MS, Devesa SS. Plasmacytoma of bone, extramedullary plasmacytoma, and multiple myeloma: incidence and survival in the United States, 1992–2004. Br J Haematol. 2009;144(1):86–94.

12. Shih LY, Dunn P, Leung WM, et al. Localised plasmacytomas in Taiwan: comparison between extramedullary plasmacytoma and solitary plasmacytoma of bone. Br J Cancer. 1995;71:128.

13. Frassica DA, Frassica FJ, Schray MF, et al. Solitary plasmacytoma of bone: Mayo Clinic experience. Int J Radiat Oncol Biol Phys. 1989;16:43.

14. McLain RF, Weinstein JN. Solitary plasmacytomas of the spine: a review of 84 cases. J Spinal Disord. 1989;2:69–74.

15. Bataille R, Sany J. Solitary myeloma: clinical and prognostic features of a review of 114 cases. Cancer. 1981;48:845.

16. Vaicys C, Schulder M, Wolansky LJ, Fromowitz FB. Falco-tentorial plasmacytoma. J Neurosurg. 1999;91:132–5.

17. Vijaya-Sekaran S, Delap T, Abramovich S. Solitary plasmacytoma of the skull base presenting with unilateral sensorineural hearing loss. J Laryngol Otol. 1999;113:164–6.

18. Burt M, Karpeh M, Ukoha O, et al. Medical tumors of the chest wall: solitary plasmacytoma and Ewing's sarcoma. J Thorac Cardiovasc Surg. 1993;105:89–96.

19. Gerry D, Lentsch EJ. Epidemiologic evidence of superior outcomes for extramedullary plasmacytoma of the head and neck. Otolaryngol Head Neck Surg. 2013;148:974.

20. Han YJ, Park SJ, Park MI, Moon W, Kim SE, Ku KH, Ock SY. Solitary extramedullary plasmacytoma in the gastrointestinal tract: report of two cases and review of literature. Korean J Gastroenterol. 2014;63(5):316–20.

21. Shaikh G, Sehgal R, Mehrishi A, Karnik A. Primary pulmonary plasmacytoma. JCO 2008;26(18):3089–91.
22. Kim SH, Kim TH, Sohn JW, Yoon HJ, Shin DH, Kim IS, Park SS. Primary pulmonary plasmacytoma presenting as multiple lung nodules. Korean J Intern Med. 2012;27(1):111–3.
23. Feng PH, Huang CC, Wang CW, Wu YK, Tsai YH. Solitary pleural plasmacytomas manifested as a massive pleural effusion without evidence of monoclonal gammopathy. Respirology. 2008;13(5):751–3.
24. Lee JY, Won JH, Kim HJ, et al. Solitary extramedullary plasmacytoma of the liver without systemic monoclonal gammopathy. J Korean Med Sci. 2007;22(4):754–7.
25. Bigé N, Arnulf B, Hummel A, Keyser ED, Royal V, Buzyn A, Fakhouri F. Urinary tract obstruction due to extramedullary plasmacytoma: report of two cases. NDT Plus. 2009;2(2):143–6.
26. Rosenberg S, Shapur N, Gofrit O, Or R. Plasmacytoma of the testis in a patient with previous multiple myeloma: is the testis a sanctuary site? JCO 2010;28(27):e456–8.
27. Shakuntala PN, Praveen SR, Shankaranand B, Rajshekar K, Umadevi K, Bafna UD. A rare case of plasmacytoma of the ovary: a case report and literature review. Ecancermedicalscience. 2013;7:288.
28. Tüting T, Bork K. Primary plasmacytoma of the skin. J Am Acad Dermatol. 1996;34(2 Pt 2):386–90.
29. Menke DM, Horny HP, Griesser H, et al. Primary lymph node plasmacytomas (plasmacytic lymphomas). Am J Clin Pathol. 2001;115:119–26.
30. Wavre A, Baur AS, Betz M, et al. Case study of intracerebral plasmacytoma as an initial presentation of multiple myeloma. Neuro Oncol. 2007;9(3):370–2.
31. Pambuccian SE, Horyd ID, Cawte T, Huvis AG. Amyloidoma of bone, a plasma cell/plasmacytoid neoplasm. Report of three cases and review of the literature. Am J Surg Pathol. 1997;21:179–86.
32. Nagasaka T, Lai R, Kuno K, Nakashima T, Nakashima N. Localised amyloidosis and extramedullary plasmacytoma involving the larynx of a child. Hum Pathol. 2001;32:132–4.
33. Kyle RA, Rajkumar SV. Criteria for diagnosis, staging, risk stratification and response assessment of multiple myeloma. Leukemia. 2009;23(1):3–9.
34. Hughes M, Soutar R, Lucraft H, Owen R, Bird J, et al. Guidelines on the diagnosis and management of solitary plasmacytoma of bone, extramedullary plasmacytoma and multiple solitary plasmacytomas: 2009 update.
35. Warsame R, Gertz MA, Lacy MQ, et al. Trends and outcomes of modern staging of solitary plasmacytoma of bone. Am J Hematol. 2012;87:647.
36. Rawstrom AC, Orfao A, et al. Report of the European Myeloma Network on multiparametric flow cytometry in multiple myeloma and related disorders. 2008;93:431–8.
37. Guidelines Working Group of the UK Myeloma Forum (UKMF). Guidelines on the diagnosis and management of solitary plasmacytoma

of bone and solitary extramedullary plasmacytoma. Br J Haematol. 2004;124:717–26.

38. Soutar R, Lucraft H, Jackson G, et al. Guidelines on the diagnosis and management of solitary plasmacytoma of bone and solitary extramedullary plasmacytoma. Clin Oncol (R Coll Radiol). 2004;16:405–13.

39. Dingli D, Kyle RA, Rajkumar SV, Nowakowski GS, Larson DR, Bida JP, Gertz MA, Therneau TM, Melton JL, Dispenzieri A, Katzmann JA. Immunoglobulin free light chains and solitary plasmacytoma of bone. Blood. 2006;108(6):1979–83.

40. Guillemette F, Guidez S, Herbaux C et al. Impact of Initial FDG-PET/CT and serum-free light chain on transformation of conventionally defined solitary plasmacytoma to multiple myeloma. Clin Cancer Res. 2014;20 (12).

41. Walker RC, Jones-Jackson LB, Rasmussen E, et al. PET and PET/CT imaging in multiple myeloma, solitary plasmacytoma, MGUS, and other plasma cell dyscrasias. Positron Emiss Tomogr. 283–302.

42. Dimopoulos MA, Hillengass J, Usmani S, et al. Role of magnetic resonance imaging in the management of patients with multiple myeloma: a consensus statement. J Clin Oncol. 2015;33:657.

43. Moulopoulos LA, Dimopoulos MA, Weber D, Fuller L, Libshitz HI, Alexanian R. Magnetic resonance imaging in the staging of solitary plasmacytoma of bone. JCO. 1993;11(7):1311–5.

44. Liebross RH, Ha CS, Cox JD, et al. Solitary bone plasmacytoma: outcome and prognostic factors following radiotherapy. Int J Radiat Oncol Biol Phys. 1998;41:1063–7.

45. Bredella MA, Steinbach L, Caputo G, et al. Value of FDG PET in the assessment of patients with multiple myeloma. AJR Am J Roentgenol. 2005;184:1199–204.

46. Lu YY, Chen JH, Lin WY, et al. FDG PET or PET/CT for detecting intramedullary and extramedullary lesions in multiple myeloma: a systematic review and meta-analysis. Clin Nucl Med. 2012;37:833–7.

47. Schrirrmeister H, Buck AK, Bergmann L, Reske SN. Positron emission tomography (PET) for staging of solitary plasmacytoma. Cancer Biother Radiopharm. 2003;18:841–5.

48. Pertuiset E, Bellaiche L, Lioté F, Laredo JD. Magnetic resonance imaging of the spine in plasma cell dyscrasias. A review. Rev Rhum Engl Ed. 1996;63:837.

49. Kim PJ, Hicks RJ, Wirth A, et al. Impact of 18F-fluorodeoxyglucose positron emission tomography before and after definitive radiation therapy in patients with apparently solitary plasmacytoma. Int J Radiat Oncol Biol Phys. 2009;74:740.

50. Nanni C, Rubello D, Zamagni E, et al. 18F-FDG PET/CT in myeloma with presumed solitary plasmocytoma of bone. In Vivo. 2008;22(4):513–7.

51. Zamagni E, Nanni C, Patriarca F, et al. A prospective comparison of 18F-fluorodeoxyglucose positron emission tomography-computed tomography, magnetic resonance imaging and whole-body planar radiographs in the assessment of bone disease in newly diagnosed multiple myeloma. Haematologica. 2007;92:50–5.

52. Salaun PY, Gastinne T, Frampas E, Bodet-Milin C, Moreau P, Bodere-Kraeber F. FDG-positron-emission tomography for staging and therapeutic assessment in patients with plasmacytoma. Haematologica Hematol J. 2008;93(8):1269–71.
53. Chak LY, Cox RS, Bostwick DG, et al. Solitary plasmacytoma of bone: treatment, progression, and survival. J Clin Oncol. 1987;5:1811–5.
54. Tsang RW, Gospodarowiez MK, Pintille M, et al. Solitary plasmacytoma treated with radio therapy: impact of tumor size on outcome. Int J Radiat Oncol Biol Phys. 2001;50:113–20.
55. Wilder RB, Ha CS, Cox JD, Weber D, Delasalle K, Alexanian R. Persistence of myeloma protein for more than one year after radiotherapy is an adverse prognostic factor in solitary plasmacytoma of bone. Cancer. 2002;94:1532–7.
56. Knobel D, Zhouhair A, Tsang RW, et al. Prognostic factors in solitary plasmacytoma of the bone: a multicenter Rare Cancer Network study. BMC Cancer. 2006;6, article 118.
57. Ozsahin M, Tsang RW, Poortmans P, et al. Outcomes and patterns of failure in solitary plasmacytoma: a multicenter rare cancer network study of 258 patients. Int J Radiat Oncol Biol Phys. 2006;64(1):210–7.
58. Kilciksiz S, Celik OK, Pak Y, et al. Clinical and prognostic features of plasmacytomas: a multicenter study of Turkish Oncology Group—Sarcoma Working Party. Am J Hematol. 2008;83(9):702–7.
59. Knowling MA, Harwood AR, Bergsagel DE. Comparison of extramedullary plasmacytomas with solitary and multiple plasma cell tumors of bone. J Clin Oncol. 1983;1:255–62.
60. Soesan M, Paccagnella A, Chiarion-Sileni V, et al. Extramedullary plasmacytoma. Clinical behaviour and response to treatment. Ann Oncol. 1992;3:51–7.
61. Liebross RH, Ha CS, Cox JD, Weber D, Delasalle K, Alexanian R. Clinical course of solitary extramedullary plasmacytoma. Radiother Oncol. 1999;52(3):245–9.
62. Strojan P, Soba E, Lamovec J, Munda A. Extramedullary plasmacytoma: clinical and histopathologic study. Int J Radiat Oncol Biol Phys. 2002;53 (3):692–701.
63. Chao MC, Gibbs P, Wirth A, Quong G, Guiney MJ, Liew KH. Radiotherapy in the management of solitary extramedullary plasmacytoma. Intern Med J. 2005;35(4):211–5.
64. Mendenhall CM, Thar TL, Million RR. Solitary plasmacytoma of bone and soft tissue. Int J Radiat Oncol Biol Phys. 1980;6:1497–501.
65. Tournier-Rangeard L, Lapeyre M, Graff-Caillaud P, Mege A, Dolivet G, Toussaint B, Charra-Brunaud C, Hoffstetter S, Marchal C, Peiffert D. Radiotherapy for solitary extramedullary plasmacytoma in the head and neck region: a dose greater than 45 Gy to the target volume improves the local control. Int J Radiat Oncol Biol Phys. 2006;64:1013–7.
66. Kilciksiz S, Karakoyun-Celik O, Agaoglu FY, Haydaroglu A, et al. A review for solitary plasmacytoma of bone and extramedullary plasmacytoma. Sci World J. 2012;Article ID 895765.
67. Alexanian R. Localized and indolent myeloma. Blood. 1980;56:521–6.

68. Fang Z, Yi X, Zhu T. Anterior approach to the second thoracic vertebral body for surgical treatment (vertebrectomy, bone grafting and titanium alloy plate fixation). Int J Clin Oncol. 2001;6:205–8.
69. Muhlbauer M, Pfisterer W, Eyb R, Knosp E. Noncontiguous spinal metastases and plasmacytomas should be operated on through a single posterior midline approach, and circumferential decompression should be performed with individualized reconstruction. Acta Neurochir (Wien). 2000;142:1219–30.
70. Jantunen E, Koivunen E, Putkonen M, et al. Autologous stem cell transplantation in patients with high risk plasmacytoma. Eur J Haematol. 2005;74:402–6.
71. Aviles A, Huerta-Guzman J, Delgado S. Improved outcome in solitary bone plasmacytomata with combined therapy. Haematol Oncol. 1996;14:111–7.
72. Holland J, Trenkner DA, Wasserman TH, Fineberg BL. Plasmacytoma. Treatment results and conversion to myeloma. Cancer. 1992;69:1513–7.
73. Delauche-Cavallier MC, Laredo JD, Wybier M, et al. Solitary plasmacytoma of the spine: long-term clinical course. Cancer. 1988;61 (8):1707–14.
74. Terpos E, Sezer O, Croucher PI, et al. The use of bisphosphonates in multiple myeloma: recommendations of an expert panel on behalf of the European Myeloma Network. Ann Oncol. 2009;20:1303–17.
75. http://www.nccn.org/professionals/physician_gls/pdf/myeloma.pdf.
76. Creach KM, Foote RL, Neben-Wittich MA, Kyle RA. Radiotherapy for extramedullary plasmacytoma of the head and neck. Int J Radiat Oncol Biol Phys. 2009;73:789.
77. Kyle RA. Monoclonal gammopathy of undetermined significance and solitary plasmacytoma: implications for progression to overt multiple myeloma. Hematology. 1997;11(1):71–87.
78. Bolek TW, Marcus RB, Mendenhall NP. Solitary plasmacytoma of bone and soft tissue. Int J Radiat Oncol Biol Phys. 1996;36(2):329–33.
79. Weber DM. Solitary bone and extramedullary plasmacytoma. Am Soc Hematol Edu Book. 2005;373–376.
80. Susnerwala SS, Shanks JH, Banerjee SS. Extramedullary plasmacytoma of the head and neck region: clinicopathological correlation in 25 cases. Br J Cancer. 1997;75(6):921–7.
81. Kumar S, Fonseca R, Dispenzieri A, et al. Prognostic value of angiogenesis in solitary bone plasmacytoma. Blood. 2003;101(5):1715–7.
82. Reed V, Shah J, Medeiros LJ, et al. Solitary plasmacytomas: outcome and prognostic factors after definitive radiation therapy. Cancer. 2011;117:4468–74.
83. Jackson A, Scarffe JH. Prognostic significance of osteopenia and immunoparesis at presentation in patients with solitary myeloma of bone. Eur J Cancer. 1990;26:363–71.
84. Mayr NA, Wen BC, Hussey DH, et al. The role of radiation therapy in the treatment of solitary plasmacytomas. Radiother Oncol. 1990;17:293–303.
85. Dimopouloos MA, Papadimitriou C, Anagnostopoulos A, Mitsibounas D, Fermand JP. High dose therapy with autologous stem cell transplantation

for solitary plasmacytoma complicated by local relapse or isolated distant recurrence. Leuk Lymphoma. 2003;44:153–5.

86. UK Myeloma Forum and the Nordic Study Group. Guidelines on the diagnosis and management of multiple myeloma. Br J Haematol. 2005;132:410–51.

Chapter 3
POEMS Syndrome and Castleman's Disease

Angela Dispenzieri, MD

POEMS Syndrome

POEMS syndrome is a rare paraneoplastic syndrome due to an underlying plasma cell disorder. Other names of the POEMS syndrome that are less frequently used are osteosclerotic myeloma, Takatsuki syndrome, or Crow–Fukase syndrome [1, 2]. The acronym, which was coined by Bardwick et al. in 1980 [3], refers to several of the features of the syndrome: polyradiculoneuropathy, organomegaly, endocrinopathy, monoclonal plasma cell disorder, and skin changes. There are other important features not included in the POEMS acronym, including *p*apilledema, *e*xtravascular volume overload, *s*clerotic bone lesions, *t*hrombocytosis/erythrocytosis (P.E.S.T.), elevated VEGF (vascular endothelial growth factor) levels, a predisposition toward thrombosis, and abnormal pulmonary function tests [4]. There is also a Castleman's disease variant of POEMS syndrome may is associated with a clonal

A. Dispenzieri, MD (✉)
Division of Hematology, Department of Medicine, Mayo Clinic,
200 First Street SW, Rochester, MN, USA
e-mail: Dispenzieri.angela@mayo.edu

© Springer Science+Business Media New York 2017
T.M. Zimmerman and S.K. Kumar (eds.),
Biology and Management of Unusual Plasma Cell Dyscrasias,
DOI 10.1007/978-1-4419-6848-7_3

plasma cell disorder. A national survey conducted in Japan in 2003 showed a prevalence of approximately 0.3 per 100,000 [5].

Pathogenesis of POEMS Syndrome

The pathogenesis of the syndrome is not well understood. To date, VEGF is the cytokine that correlates best with disease activity [6, 7], although it may not be the driving force of the disease based on the mixed results seen with anti-VEGF therapy [8]. VEGF is known to target endothelial cells, induce a rapid and reversible increase in vascular permeability, and be important in angiogenesis. It is expressed by osteoblasts, in bone tissue, macrophages, tumor cells (including plasma cells), and megakaryocytes/platelets. Both IL-1β and IL-6 have been shown to stimulate VEGF production [9]. IL-12 has also been shown to correlate with disease activity [10], and other pro-angiogenetic factors have been implicated [11]. Recently, N-terminal propeptide of type I collagen has been described as a novel marker for the diagnosis of patients with POEMS [12].

Little is known about the plasma cells in POEMS syndrome except that more than 95 % of the time they are lambda light chain restricted with restricted immunoglobulin light chain variable gene usage (IGLV1) [4]. Translocations and deletion of chromosome 13 have been described, but hyperdiploidy is not seen.

Diagnosis of POEMS Syndrome

The diagnosis is made based on a composite of clinical and laboratory features which are listed in Table 3.1 along with their estimated frequencies. Most notably, the constellation of neuropathy and any of the following should elicit an in depth search for POEMS syndrome: thrombocytosis [13], monoclonal protein (especially lambda light chain), anasarca, or papilledema. Any patient who carries a diagnosis of chronic inflammatory demyelinating polyneuropathy (CIDP) that is not responding to standard CIDP therapy should be considered as a possible POEMS syndrome patient. Helpful cutoffs for plasma and serum VEGF levels to diagnosis POEMS syndrome are 200 pg/mL (specificity 95 %; sensitivity 68 %) [7] and 1920 pg/mL (specificity 98 %; sensitivity 73 %) [12], respectively.

Distinctive presenting characteristics of the syndrome that differentiate POEMS syndrome from standard multiple myeloma (MM) include the following: (1) dominant symptoms are typically neuropathy, endocrine dysfunction, and volume overload (2); dominant symptoms have little to nothing to do with bone pain, extremes of bone marrow infiltration by plasma cells, or renal failure; (3) VEGF levels are high; (4) sclerotic bone lesions are present in the majority of cases; (5) overall survival is typically superior; and (6) lambda clones predominate [14].

The neuropathy is the dominant characteristic. The neuropathy is peripheral, ascending, symmetrical, and affecting both sensation and motor function [15]; in our experience, pain may be a dominant feature in about 10–15 % of patients, and in one report, as many as 76 % of patients had hyperesthesia [5, 16]. Patients are typically areflexic, and they have steppage gait. Nerve conduction studies in patients with POEMS syndrome show slowing of nerve conduction that is more predominant in the intermediate than distal nerve segments as compared to CIDP, and there is more severe attenuation of compound muscle action potentials in the lower than upper limbs [5, 17]. In contrast to CIDP, conduction block is rare. Axonal loss is greater in POEMS syndrome than it is in CIDP [17].

Endocrinopathy is a central but poorly understood feature of POEMS. On examination, gynecomastia and darkened areolae may be seen. In a recent series [18], approximately 84 % of patients had a recognized endocrinopathy, with hypogonadism as the most common endocrine abnormality, followed by thyroid abnormalities, glucose metabolism abnormalities, and lastly by adrenal insufficiency. The majority of patients have evidence of multiple endocrinopathies in the four major endocrine axes (gonadal, thyroid, glucose, and adrenal).

The monoclonal plasma cell disorder is most typically characterized by a small IgA lambda or IgG lambda found in the serum by immunofixation. In a minority of cases, the monoclonal plasma cell disorder is only found by biopsying one of the sclerotic or mixed lytic sclerotic bone lesions or by iliac crest bone marrow aspirate and biopsy. The one-third of patients who do not have

Table 3.1 Criteria for the diagnosis of POEMS syndrome

Criteria	Individual criterion	% affected
Mandatory major (both required)	1. Polyneuropathy (typically demyelinating)	100
	2. Monoclonal plasma cell-proliferative disorder (almost always λ)	100
Other major (one required)	3. Castleman's disease[a]	11–25
	4. Sclerotic bone lesions	27–97
	5. Vascular endothelial growth factor elevation	
Minor	6. Organomegaly (splenomegaly, hepatomegaly, or lymphadenopathy)	45–85
	7. Extravascular volume overload (edema, pleural effusion, or ascites)	29–87
	8. Endocrinopathy (adrenal, thyroid,[b] pituitary, gonadal, parathyroid, pancreatic[b])	67–84
	9. Skin changes (hyperpigmentation, hypertrichosis, glomeruloid hemangiomata, plethora, acrocyanosis, flushing, white nails)	68–89
	10. Papilledema	29–64
	11. Thrombocytosis/polycythemia[c]	54–88
Other symptoms and signs	Clubbing, weight loss, hyperhidrosis, pulmonary hypertension/restrictive lung disease, thrombotic diatheses, diarrhea, low vitamin B_{12} values	

POEMS, polyneuropathy, organomegaly, endocrinopathy, M-protein, skin changes. The diagnosis of POEMS syndrome is confirmed when both of the mandatory major criteria, one of the three other major criteria, and one of the six minor criteria are present

[a]There is a Castleman's disease variant of POEMS syndrome that occurs *without* evidence of a clonal plasma cell disorder that is not accounted for in this table. This entity should be considered separately

[b]Because of the high prevalence of diabetes mellitus and thyroid abnormalities, this diagnosis alone is not sufficient to meet this minor criterion

[c]Approximately 50 % of patients will have bone marrow changes that distinguish it from a typical MGUS or myeloma bone marrow [19]. Anemia and/or thrombocytopenia are distinctively unusual in this syndrome unless Castleman's disease is present

Taken with permission from [4]

clonal plasma cells on their iliac crest biopsy are the patients who present at with a solitary or "multiple solitary plasmacytomas." Two-thirds of patients have clonal plasma cells on bone marrow biopsy, and 91 % of these cases are clonal lambda. The median percent of plasma cells observed is less than 5 %. Immunohistochemical staining is more sensitive than is 6-color flow since the former provides information on bone marrow architecture, which is key in making the diagnosis in nearly half of cases. In our study of pretreatment bone marrows biopsies from patients with POEMS syndrome, lymphoid aggregates were found in 49 % of cases. Of these, there was plasma cell rimming in all but one, and in 75 and 4 %, the rimming was clonal lambda and kappa, respectively. This finding was not seen in bone marrows from normal controls or from patients with MGUS, multiple myeloma, or amyloidosis. Megakaryocyte hyperplasia and megakaryocyte clustering are observed in 54 and 93 %, respectively, of patient's bone marrows [19]. These megakaryocyte findings are reminiscent of a myeloproliferative disorder, but *JAK2*V617F mutation is uniformly absent. Overall, only 8/67 (12 %) of POEMS cases had normal iliac crest bone marrow biopsies, i.e., no detectable clonal plasma cells, no plasma cell rimmed lymphoid aggregates, and no megakaryocyte hyperplasia.

Skin examination may reveal hyperpigmentation, a recent out-cropping of hemangioma, hypertrichosis, dependent rubor and acrocyanosis, white nails, sclerodermoid changes, facial atrophy, flushing, or clubbing (Fig. 3.1). Rarely calciphylaxis is also seen.

Papilledema is present in at least one-third of patients (Fig. 3.1) [20, 21]. The most common ocular symptoms reported were blurred vision in 15, diplopia in 5, and ocular pain in 3. In one series, papilledema was an adverse prognostic feature for overall survival [21].

After neuropathy, the next most disabling feature is the extravascular overload. Extravascular overload most commonly manifests as peripheral edema, but pleural effusion, ascites, and pericardial effusions are also common. Recalcitrant ascites and effusions are not common, but can be disabling and lead to pre-renal azotemia. Based on low serum ascites albumin gradients, the fluid is exudative in 74 % of cases [22].

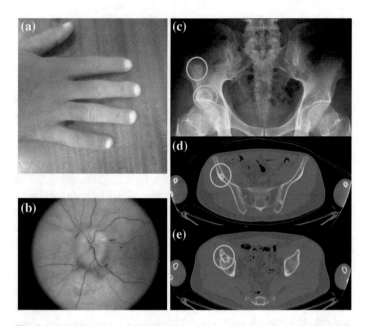

Fig. 3.1 Manifestations of POEMS syndrome skin changes including white nails and cyanosis optic disk edema **c–e**. Mixed lytic osteosclerotic bone lesions on plain radiograph (**c**) and CT scan (**d** and **e**). Taken with permission from [4]

Osteosclerotic (or mixed lytic and osteosclerotic) lesions occur in approximately 95 % of patients and can be confused with benign bone islands, aneurysmal bone cysts, non-ossifying fibromas, and fibrous dysplasia [2, 23]. Some lesions are densely sclerotic, while others are lytic with a sclerotic rim and still others have a mixed soap-bubble appearance (Fig. 3.1). Bone windows of CT body images are often very informative, often even more so than FDG uptake, which can be variable [24, 25]. FDG uptake occurs in those lesions which have a lytic component. The advantage of whole body CT—even low dose like what is quickly becoming the standard in multiple myeloma—is that other features of the disease are also seen: effusions, ascites, adenopathy, and hepatosplenomegaly.

Laboratory findings are notable for an absence of cytopenias. In fact, nearly half of patients will have thrombocytosis or erythrocytosis [23]. In the series of Li and colleagues, 26 % of patients had anemia, which the authors attributed to impaired renal function [26]. Their series was enriched with Castleman's disease cases (25 %), which may have also contributed to this unprecedentedly high rate of anemia.

Patients are at increased risk for arterial and/or venous thromboses during their course, with nearly 20 % of patients experiencing one of these complications [14, 27]. Ten percent of patients present with a cerebrovascular event, most commonly embolic or vessel dissection and stenosis [28]. Risk factors for cerebral events included thrombocytosis and bone marrow plasmacytosis. Aberrations in the coagulation cascade have been implicated in POEMS syndrome [29].

Plasma and serum levels of VEGF are markedly elevated in patients with POEMS [7, 9, 30] and correlate with the activity of the disease [7, 9, 31, 32]. VEGF levels are independent of M-protein size [31]. Other diseases with high VEGF include connective tissue disease and vasculitis [7].

Respiratory complaints are usually limited given patients' neurologic status impairing their ability to induce cardiovascular challenges [33]. The pulmonary manifestations are protean, including pulmonary hypertension, restrictive lung disease, impaired neuromuscular respiratory function, and impaired diffusion capacity of carbon monoxide, but improve with effective therapy [33, 34]. Pulmonary hypertension has been reported to occur in 27 % of unselected patients with POEMS syndrome [35]. It is more likely to occur in patients with extravascular overload. Whether the digital clubbing seen in POEMS is a reflection of underlying pulmonary hypertension and/or parenchymal disease is yet to be determined. Impaired DLCO has been shown to be an adverse prognostic factor another series [21].

Serum creatinine levels are normal in most cases, but serum cystatin C, which is a surrogate marker for renal function, is high in 71 % of patients [36]. In our experience, at presentation, fewer than 10 % of patients have proteinuria exceeding 0.5 g/24 h, and only 6 % have a serum creatinine greater than or equal to 1.5 mg/dL. Four percent of patients developed renal failure as preterminal events [23]. In another series from China, 22 % of patients had a creatinine clearance (CrCl) of less than 60 ml/min/m^2 [37]. In our experience, renal disease is more likely to occur in patients who have coexisting Castleman's disease.

POEMS Syndrome Risk Stratification

To date, there are no known molecular or genetic risk factors that predict for overall survival. The course of POEMS syndrome is usually chronic with modern estimated median survivals of nearly 14 years [23, 33]. Only fingernail clubbing, extravascular volume overload—i.e., effusions, edema, and ascites [23], respiratory symptoms [33], pulmonary hypertension [35] impaired DLCO, and papilledema [21]—have been associated with a significantly shorter overall survival. The number of POEMS features does not affect survival [14, 38]. Patients who are candidates for radiation therapy have a better overall survival (Fig. 3.2) [23]. Patients with coexisting Castleman's disease may have an inferior overall survival as compared to patients without [26]. In a series of 11 patients, lower VEGF levels predicted for better response to therapy, with resolution of the skin changes, improvement of the neuropathic disturbances, and reduction all of the features assumed to be related to increased permeability, like papilledema and organomegaly [32]. Thrombocytosis and increased bone marrow infiltration are associated with risk for cerebrovascular accidents [28].

POEMS Syndrome Therapy Overview

Despite the relationship between disease response and dropping levels of VEGF, the most experience with successful outcomes has been associated with directing therapy at the underlying clonal plasma cell disorder rather than solely targeting VEGF with anti-VEGF antibodies. The treatment algorithm is based on the extent of the plasma cell infiltration (Fig. 3.2). There are those patients who do not have bone marrow involvement as determined by blind iliac crest sampling and those who do have disseminated disease, i.e., either bone diffuse marrow involvement and/or more than 3 skeletal lesions, and the approach to these 2 groups of patients differs.

Treating Isolated Plasmacytomas

In the case of patients with an isolated bone lesion without clonal plasma cells found on iliac crest biopsy, radiation is the recommended therapy as it is in the case of a more straightforward solitary plasmacytoma of bone. Not only does radiation to an isolated (or even two or three isolated) lesion(s) improve the symptoms of POEMS syndrome over the course of 3–36 months, but it can be curative with a 4-year overall survival of 97 % and a 4-year failure-free survival of 52 % [39]. More than half the "failures" occur within 12 months of radiation. Whether these were true failures or whether they were driven by patient and physician anxiety over slow response is unclear in this retrospective series.

Treating a Disseminated Clone

Once there is disseminated bone marrow involvement, albeit even with a low plasma cell percentage, radiation is not expected to be curative, and systemic therapy is recommended with the caveat that large bony lesions with a significant lytic component may require adjuvant radiation therapy. Decisions about adjuvant radiation should be made on a case by case basis. Optimal FDG-PET response may also lag by 6–12 months after completing chemotherapy. There is a lag between completion of successful therapy and neurologic response, often with no discernible improvement until 6 months after completion of therapy. Maximal response is not seen until 2–3 years hence. Other features like anasarca, papilledema, and even skin changes may improve sooner.

Since there are no published randomized clinical trials among patients with POEMS syndrome, treatment recommendations are largely based on case series and anecdote. The treatment armamentarium is borrowed from other plasma cell disorders, most notably multiple myeloma and light chain amyloidosis. Table 3.2

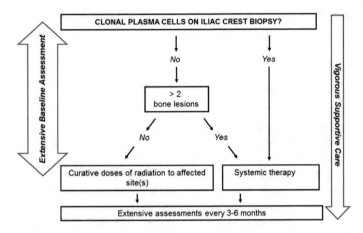

Fig. 3.2 Algorithm for the treatment of POEMS syndrome [4]

demonstrates a summary of observed outcomes. Corticosteroids may provide symptomatic improvement, but response duration is limited. The most experience has been with alkylator-based therapy, either low dose or high dose with peripheral blood stem cell transplant. The first prospective clinical trial to treat POEMS syndrome included 31 patients who were treated with 12 cycles of melphalan and dexamethasone [40]. Eighty-one percent of patients had hematologic response, 100 % had VEGF response, and 100 % with at least some improvement in neurologic status. A limitation of this study is that follow-up was only 21 months, so long-term outcomes are not yet available. Personal experience and retrospective reports of the use of cyclophosphamide-based therapy are also promising.

The French have reported in abstract form their results of a Phase 2 study of lenalidomide and dexamethasone for 2 cycles as neoadjuvant therapy preceding radiation or high-dose therapy or as primary therapy as 9 cycles followed by 12 cycles of single-agent lenalidomide [41]. They have treated 27 patients: 10 pre-radiation therapy; 8 pre-ASCT; and 9 as primary therapy. Although follow-up is short, the authors report that several patients had rapid neurologic response, no patient has died, and 1 patient has progressed. These results are similar to previous case reports and case series [42–44] though relapses have been reported. In the largest case series of 20 patients [44], all patients responded, but 4 patients relapsed 3–10 months after the end of treatment. Three of these treatment failures responded to further therapy, including one who responded to reintroduction of the lenalidomide–dexamethasone combination. A systematic review of lenalidomide use in patients with POEMS has been published [45]. Given the intrinsic risk patients with POEMS syndrome have for thrombosis, it is imperative that at least an aspirin be used for prophylaxis. The use of low molecular weight heparin or warfarin should be balanced against fall risk.

Thalidomide in combination with dexamethasone has also shown to produce responses in terms of VEGF, peripheral neuropathy, and extravascular volume overload, but hematologic responses have not been reported [46]. Enthusiasm for this therapy should be tempered by the risk of peripheral neuropathy induced by this drug. The Japanese are accruing to a randomized trial of thalidomide plus dexamethasone versus dexamethasone alone [47].

Like lenalidomide and thalidomide, bortezomib also has anti-VEGF and anti-TNF effects. Bortezomib use has been reported in 5 patients with excellent response [4]. Enthusiasm for the bortezomib and/or thalidomide should be tempered by their risk of drug induced peripheral neuropathy.

High-dose chemotherapy with peripheral blood stem cell transplant can also be quite effective, but selection basis may confound these reports. Case series suggest 100 % of patients achieve at least some neurologic improvement [8, 48, 49]. Doses of melphalan ranging from 140 to 200 mg/m^2 have been used, with the lower doses used for sicker patients. In addition, tandem transplant has been applied in one patient, but again, no information is available regarding any added value of the second transplant [50]. Of the 59 patients with POEMS syndrome treated at the Mayo Clinic Rochester, progression-free survival was 98, 94, and 75 % at 1, 2, and 5 years, respectively [48]. Treatment-related morbidity and mortality can minimized by recognizing and treating an engraftment-type syndrome characterized by fevers, rash, diarrhea, weight gain, and respiratory symptoms and signs that occurs anytime between days 7 and 15 post-stem cell infusion [51]. A starting dose of prednisone ranging between 20 and 1500 mg/day has been used.

Although an anti-VEGF strategy is appealing, the results with bevacizumab have been mixed, and its use is not recommended [4, 8].

Both our experience and the literature would support that single-agent intravenous gammaglobulin (IVIG) or plasmapheresis is not helpful. A recent report, however, describes reduction in serum VEGF and clinical improvement with single-agent IVIG. The response was not durable, which prompted another course of IVIG with radiation to a solitary plasmacytoma [52]. Other treatments like interferon-alpha, tamoxifen, trans-retinoic acid,

Table 3.2 Activity of therapy for the treatment of POEMS syndrome

Regimen	Outcome
Radiation	50–70 % of patients have significant clinical improvement
Melphalan–dexamethasone	81 % hematologic response rate; 100 % with some neurologic improvement
Corticosteroids	50 % of patients have significant clinical improvement
Cyclophosphamide–dexamethasone	At least 50 % of patients have significant improvement
ASCT	100 % of surviving patients have significant clinical improvement
Thalidomide–dexamethasone	Reported responses in 12 patients, but not recommended as first line due to risk of neuropathy
Lenalidomide–dexamethasone	Reported responses in majority of patients (more than 60 patients reported)
Bortezomib	Used as single agent ($n = 1$), with dexamethasone ($n = 2$), with cyclophosphamide and dexamethasone ($n = 1$), and with doxorubicin and dexamethasone ($n = 1$). Reported responses in all
Bevacizumab	Two out of 3 using it as single agent died within weeks; one improved. Two other patients using it as "salvage" improved, but relapsed and died despite continued therapy, normal VEGF at 3.5 and 5.5 years. Six other cases of use with or after other alkylator-based therapy yielded one death and 4 patients with improvement

Taken with permission from [4]

ticlopidine, argatroban, and strontium-89 have been reported as having activity mostly as single case reports [14].

Supportive Care, Response, and Follow-up

Attention to supportive care is imperative. Orthotics, physical therapy, and CPAP all play an important role in patients' recovery. Ankle foot orthotics can increase mobility and reduce falls. Physical therapy reduces the risk for permanent contractures and leads to improved function both in the long and short term. For those with severe neuromuscular weakness, CPAP and/or biBAP provides better oxygenation and potentially reduces the risk complications associated with hypoventilation like pulmonary infection and pulmonary hypertension. Patients should also be screened for depression [53].

Patients must be followed carefully every 3–6 months tracking the status of deficits comparing these to baseline [48]. VEGF responses may occur as soon as 3 months [54], but they can be delayed. VEGF is an imperfect marker since discordance between disease activity and response have been reported, so trends rather than absolute values should direct therapeutic decisions. Serum M-protein responses by protein electrophoresis, immunofixation electrophoresis, or serum immunoglobulin free light chains also pose a challenge. The size of the M-protein is typically small making standard multiple myeloma response criteria inapplicable in most cases. In addition, patients can derive very significant clinical benefit in the absence of and M-protein response [51, 55]. Finally, despite the fact that the immunoglobulin free light chains are elevated in 67–90 % of POEMS patients, the ratio is normal in all but 13–18 % [36, 56], making the test of limited value for patients with POEMS syndrome.

Recommendations about how to approach organ response have recently been suggested for the purposes of clinical trials since there are more than 2-dozen parameters that can be assessed in a given patient with POEMS syndrome given the multisystem nature of the disease [48, 57]. Alternatively, response criteria for POEMS syndrome could be abridged as follows: (1) hematologic response using a modified amyloid response criteria; (2) VEGF response; (3) and a simplified organ response, which is limited to those systems causing the most morbidity, like peripheral neuropathy assessment, pulmonary function testing (diffusion capacity of carbon monoxide), and extravascular overload (grading ascites and pleural effusion as absent, mild, moderate, or severe).

Castleman's Disease

Castleman's disease (CD) was first described in the 1950s as localized mediastinal lymph node enlargement characterized by redundancy of lymphoid follicles with germinal-center involution and marked capillary proliferation, including follicular and inter-follicular endothelial hyperplasia [58]. Definitions have evolved over the decades, and the most commonly accepted classifications relate to HIV- and HHV-8-associated disease [59]; whether the disease is unicentric versus multicentric; and whether the pathology demonstrates the hyaline variant or the plasma cell variant. There is typically overlap between the hyaline vascular variant and localized or unicentric disease and between the plasma cell variant and disseminated or multicentric disease.

Among patients with CD, there is no gender preference, and the age distribution is bimodal with unifocal patients being in their 4th decade versus patients with multicentric disease in their 6th decade [60–62]. CD can also occur in the pediatric population [63]. With the acquired immunodeficiency syndrome (AIDS) epidemic, the incidence increased [64]; but even in this population, it is a rare condition with MCD accounting for fewer than 2 % of lymph node biopsies in human immunodeficiency virus 1 (HIV)-infected patients [65].

Pathogenesis

The pathogenesis of CD is not understood. Most have speculated that CD is a chronic inflammatory or immunologic process in reaction to an unknown stimulus [58, 66]. Nearly all HIV infection-associated MCD cases are associated with HHV-8, and nearly half of those MCD cases in patients without HIV are HHV-8 associated [67–70] HHV-8 is not associated with localized (unicentric) CD [87].

Overproduction of circulating cytokines has been implicated in the pathogenesis and symptomatology of MCD and the related entity POEMS syndrome. Serum levels of IL-6 in CD patients are significantly higher than those found in patients with lymphoid malignancies [71]. Overexpression of IL-6 in mice produces a phenotype similar to the MCD phenotype [72]. VEGF is also elevated in CD patients, but less so than in patients with POEMS syndrome [71].

Histopathology

Histopathology of Hyaline Vascular Variant

On gross examination these lesions tend to be large, single, rounded, encapsulated masses—more commonly found in central than peripheral lymph node regions. HV-CD usually involves a lymph node or a group of lymph nodes [60, 66]. Most masses are between 5 and 10 cm, though lesions as big as 25 cm have been described. On microscopic examination, the hyaline vascular variant is characterized by capsular fibrosis with broad fibrous bands traversing through the lymph node, an increased number of lymphoid follicles scattered throughout cortex and medulla with often more than one germinal center sharing the same mantle (so-called twinning). Mantles tend to be broad and composed by concentric rings of small lymphoid cells ("onion skin pattern") imparting a target-like appearance to the follicle. Often the germinal centers are depleted of small lymphoid cells and are predominantly composed of dendritic cells with prominent hyaline deposits (PAS positive). Sclerotic blood vessels penetrating within the germinal centers forming so-called lollipop lesions are observed. Dendritic cells within these depleted germinal centers can show dysplastic features. The interfollicular region is composed by prominent high endothelial venules with plump endothelial cells, often surrounded by clusters of plasmacytoid dendritic cells and stromal proliferation. Plasma cells, immunoblasts, and eosinophils are also part of the interfollicular infiltrate; however, sheets of plasma cells, as seen in the plasma cell variant, are not seen [66, 73, 74].

Histopathology of Plasma Cell Variant

Gross examination often reveals multiple discrete lymph nodes, comprising the clinically observed "mass," in contrast to the single rounded mass that is typically seen with the hyaline vascular variant; however, single masses may also be observed [60, 66]. Microscopically, the plasma cell variant is distinguished by the presence of sheets of plasma cells in the interfollicular zone [66]. The interfollicular region typically contains prominent high endothelial venules, similar to cases of hyaline vascular CD. Cases that contain mature plasma cells without increased vascularity have been included within this entity, but care is needed to rule out other causes of plasmacytosis, such as chronic inflammation or autoimmune disease. There is follicular hyperplasia with sharply defined mantles, polarized germinal centers, with frequent mitosis, and histiocytes with nuclear debris.

Mixed Variant Histopathology

Lymph nodes may have characteristics of both the hyaline vascular and plasma cell variants. Focal accumulations of plasma cells next to extensive areas without plasma cells are found in the interfollicular tissue. Characteristic lymphoid follicles with normal reactive germinal centers and regressed germinal centers are found in small areas.

Diagnosis

The diagnosis of CD is histologic though treatment algorithms are driven by HIV status and by extent of disease (unicentric versus multicentric) [59, 75]. Although HIV-associated CD is beyond the scope of this chapter, a few important points will be highlighted. CD associated with HIV differs from CD without HIV infection in the following ways: (1) it is more likely to be multicentric; (2) systemic symptoms are more common and more intense; (3) lymphadenopathy is more likely to be peripheral; (4) pulmonary symptoms are more prevalent; (5) leukopenia and thrombocytopenia are more common; (6) HHV-8 infection is virtually always present, often with clinical Kaposi's sarcoma; (7) the histologic type is most commonly the mixed HV/PC variant; (8) there is a 15-fold increased risk of developing overt malignant lymphoma; and (9) prognosis is dismal, with a median survival of 12–22 months [65, 76, 77].

Once a diagnosis of CD is made, besides a thorough examination and review of systems patients should have a complete blood count, erythrocyte sedimentation rate, C-reactive protein, liver function tests, serum creatinine, serum protein electrophoresis with immunofixation, interleukin-6, VEGF, serology for HHV-8 and HIV, urinalysis, CT chest abdomen and pelvis. If there are any pulmonary symptoms, the threshold for performing pulmonary function tests should be low. If there is associated neuropathy, imaging of the bones should be done looking for sclerotic bone lesions. If elements of POEMS syndrome present, then more extensive endocrine testing should also be performed.

Diagnosis of Unicentric Castleman's Disease

Nearly 90 % of patients with unicentric disease have the hyaline vascular morphology. These patients often present with either compressive symptoms or a large incidental mass; however, nearly 40 % of patients with localized CD have associated systemic symptoms (Table 3.3), which promptly resolve after surgical extirpation of the solitary mass. Unicentric disease occurs most commonly in the mediastinum, cervical regions, and abdominal/pelvic cavity, but nasopharyngeal, orbital, dural, and oral occurrences have been described. Solitary subdiaphragmatic CD is often of the plasma cell variant and associated with systemic symptoms. Laboratory tests may be completely normal, but anemia, hypergammaglobulinemia, and elevated sedimentation rate and liver function tests may be present, all of which promptly resolves after successful surgical removal of the mass.

Diagnosis of Multicentric Castleman's Disease

About 90 % of cases of MCD are the plasma cell variant. Approximately 80 % of patients with the plasma cell or the mixed variant have associated systemic symptoms, most commonly fatigue, fevers, night sweats, and weight loss (Table 3.3). Hepatomegaly and/or splenomegaly occur in 75 % of patients. Laboratory abnormalities are common, including anemia, low ferritin levels, elevations of the sedimentation rate, antinuclear antibodies, fibrinogen, C-reactive protein, and liver transaminases, and an abnormal urinalysis.

Paraneoplastic Symptoms and Syndromes

There are number of paraneoplastic symptoms/syndromes also associated with CD, more commonly with the multicentric form [75, 78, 79]. These include pleural effusions, pericardial effusions, ascites, anasarca, autoimmune hemolytic anemia, immune thrombocytopenic purpura, a multitude of renal disorders including secondary (AA) amyloidosis or membranoproliferative glomerulonephritis, pulmonary abnormalities ranging from infiltrates to restrictive lung disease to lymphoid interstitial pneumonitis to bronchiolitis obliterans and skin abnormalities ranging from rash to hyperpigmentation to paraneoplastic pemphigus to Bechet's disease to Kaposi's sarcoma. In one series over the course of the disease, 40 % of patients developed CNS signs, including seizures and aphasia [78]. This finding should be tempered by the fact that a number of cases from the 1980s may have been AIDS-associated CD, which is known to have a particularly dismal prognosis [65]. Neuropathy occurs in nearly 10 % of patients, again more commonly those with multicentric disease, but is also possible in patients with unicentric disease. When neuropathy is present, other features of POEMS syndrome should be sought including a monoclonal protein and osteosclerotic bone lesions [75, 80, 81].

Relationship of POEMS Syndrome to Castleman's Disease and Castleman's Disease Variant of POEMS

Several published cases of "interesting features" associated with Castleman's disease are likely cases of POEMS syndrome [75]. MCD with and without peripheral neuropathy tend to be different; it has even been proposed that the presence or absence of peripheral neuropathy should be part of the multicentric Castleman's disease classification system [73]. Those patients with peripheral neuropathy are more likely to have edema and impaired peripheral circulation, and they are also more likely to have a monoclonal lambda protein in their serum and/or urine [80].

Between 11 and 30 % of POEMS patients who have a documented clonal plasma, cell disorder also have documented Castleman's disease or Castleman-like histology [14]. In 30 patients with POEMS syndrome, 19 of 32 biopsied lymph nodes showed angiofollicular hyperplasia typical of Castleman's disease [2]. In another series, 25 of 43 biopsied lymph nodes were diagnostic of Castleman's disease and 84 % of these had hyaline vascular type [26]. Only those with peripheral neuropathy and a plasma cell clone should classified as having standard POEMS syndrome. Without both of these characteristics, patients can be classified as Castleman's disease variant of POEMS if they have other POEMS features (Fig. 3.3).

The neuropathy in Castleman's disease patients tends to be more subtle than that of POEMS patients with osteosclerotic myeloma and is more often sensory. At its worst, however, it is a mixture of demyelination and axonal degeneration with normal myelin spacing on electron microscopy [82], and abnormal capillary proliferation, similar to what is seen in the affected lymph nodes, has been described. In contrast to the osteosclerotic myeloma variant of POEMS in which VEGF is the most consistently elevated cytokine, in Castleman's disease, IL-6 is the dominant

Table 3.3 Clinical features of Castleman's disease (angiofollicular lymph node hyperplasia)

	Unicentric CD	Multicentric CD
Age	4th decade	6th decade
Symptoms	Incidental or compressive; occasional systemic symptoms	Fever, sweats, weight loss, malaise, autoimmune manifestations; may be associated with peripheral neuropathy and POEMS syndrome
LA	Central (mediastinal, abdominal) most common	Peripheral plus central
Organomegaly	Rare	Yes
Laboratory abnormalities	Occasional. Anemia, hypergammaglobulinemia, increased ESR, CRP	Common. Anemia, thrombocytopenia, hypergammaglobulinemia, increased ESR, CRP, abnormal LFTs, low albumin, renal dysfunction
Autoimmune phenomena	Rare	Often
Pathologic features	Usually hyaline vascular variant	Usually plasma cell variant
Associations with infection	No HIV or HHV-8	Some HIV and HHV-8
Therapy	Surgery; occasionally radiation if inoperable	Assorted systemic therapies with variable success (see text)
Clinical course	Benign	Usually aggressive

Abbreviations POEMS peripheral neuropathy, organomegaly, endocrinopathy, monoclonal protein, and skin changes; *CRP* C-reactive protein, *ESR* erythrocyte sedimentation rate; *LFTs* liver function tests. Taken with permission from [75] aberrantly overexpressed cytokine. Castleman's disease patients often have a brisk polyclonal hypergammaglobulinemia.

Course and Prognosis

The course of CD is variable. Typically cases of localized disease are cured by surgical resection. The multicentric form is more difficult to manage, and median survival has been reported to be as short as 26 months [83]. Frizzera et al. [78] divided patients' courses into 2 categories—episodic and persistent. Those patients with more extensive disease (systemic symptoms, lymphadenopathy, hepatosplenomegaly, and effusions) were more likely to have the episodic pattern of evolution. These authors also found that male gender, episodic evolution, and predominantly proliferative morphology in involved lymph nodes were associated with worse survival in univariate analysis [78]. Weisenberger et al. [83] described parsed the course for multicentric CD patients into five categories: (1) cure; (2) stable and persistent; (3) relapse and remission; (4) rapidly fatal disease; and (5) evolution to malignant lymphoma.

A prognostic model for survival was developed using the clinical information of 113 patients with CD who were not known to have HIV [84]. Sixty patients had multicentric disease. Of the patients with multicentric CD, 32 % had criteria sufficient for a diagnosis of POEMS syndrome. For all patients, 2, 5, and 10-year OS rates were 92, 76, 59 %, respectively. Most of the factors identified as risk factors for death on univariate analysis cosegregated with diagnostic criteria for POEMS syndrome, which supported the concept of four categories of CD, which are (along with their 5-year OS): (1) unicentric CD (91 %); (2) multicentric CD associated with the osteosclerotic variant of POEMS syndrome (90 %); (3); multicentric CD without POEMS syndrome (65 %); and (4) multicentric CD with POEMS syndrome without osteosclerotic lesions (27 %).

Secondary malignancies are not uncommon in CD. HIV-infected patients with HHV-8+ MCD are estimated to have a frequency of lymphoma of 15-fold compared to an HIV-infected population without CD [76]. HIV-negative patients with HHV-8+

MCD develop malignancies, most notably lymphoma (~ 15 %) and Kaposi sarcoma, in up to 1/3 of the cases [78].

Therapy

Treatment options will only be discussed for HIV-negative patients.

Treatment of Unicentric CD

The treatment decision for unicentric disease, regardless of whether it is hyaline vascular, plasma cell variant, or mixed type, is straightforward: surgical removal whenever possible; if not possible, irradiation should be considered [75]. For large tumors, embolization of solitary mass prior to surgical removal or neoadjuvant therapy has also been applied. Though there is a low rate of recurrence, these patients appear to have a higher risk of developing Hodgkin disease and non-Hodgkin lymphoma. A number of patients have seemingly done well with observation alone, but one must be vigilant about subtle development and progression of associated paraneoplastic entities like bronchiolitis obliterans.

Of the 22 patients with unicentric disease treated with irradiation that have been reported in the literature, 11 had a complete response, 4 had a partial response, 6 had no clinical response, and one had progressive disease [75].

When there are paraneoplastic or autoimmune conditions associated with CD, these generally resolve within months of the surgery, though the reports of resolution of associated pemphigus and bronichiolitis obliterans are mixed.

Treatment of Multicentric CD

The best choice of therapy for multicentric CD is uncertain [75]. Historically, therapy had been corticosteroid and alkylator based.

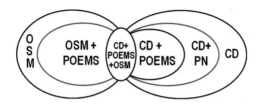

Fig. 3.3 Spectrum of disease: osteosclerotic myeloma (OSM) to POEMS to Castleman's disease (CD). Taken with permission from Blood Reviews. 2007;21(6):285–99

Small numbers of patients have been treated with alternative therapies like interferon-alpha, thalidomide, rituximab, bortezomib, and high-dose chemotherapy with hematopoietic stem cell transplantation (Table 3.3) [59, 75]. The most exciting therapeutic strategies are those that block IL-6 either as an anti-IL-6 antibody or as an anti-IL-6 receptor antibody. The former approach has an FDA-approved drug, siltuximab, which produced durable tumor and symptomatic responses in 34 % of patients treated as compared to placebo for whom there were no responses [85]. The anti-IL-6 receptor approach has been used in Japan form more than a decade [86].

Acknowledgments AD and this work are support in part by the Robert A. Kyle Hematologic Malignancies Fund, the Predolin Foundation, the JABBS Foundation, and the Andrew & Lillian A. Posey Foundation.

References

1. Takatsuki K, Sanada I. Plasma cell dyscrasia with polyneuropathy and endocrine disorder: clinical and laboratory features of 109 reported cases. Jpn J Clin Oncol. 1983;13(3):543–55.
2. Nakanishi T, Sobue I, Toyokura Y, et al. The Crow-Fukase syndrome: a study of 102 cases in Japan. Neurology. 1984;34(6):712–20.
3. Bardwick PA, Zvaifler NJ, Gill GN, Newman D, Greenway GD, Resnick DL. Plasma cell dyscrasia with polyneuropathy, organomegaly, endocrinopathy, M protein, and skin changes: the POEMS syndrome. Report on two cases and a review of the literature. Medicine. 1980;59 (4):311–22.

4. Dispenzieri A. POEMS syndrome: update on diagnosis, risk-stratification, and management. American Journal of Hematology. 2015;90(10):951–62. Prepublished on 04 Sept 2015 as doi:10.1002/ajh.24171.
5. Nasu S, Misawa S, Sekiguchi Y, et al. Different neurological and physiological profiles in POEMS syndrome and chronic inflammatory demyelinating polyneuropathy. Journal of Neurology, Neurosurgery, and Psychiatry. 2012;83(5):476–79. Prepublished on 18 Feb 2012 as doi:10.1136/jnnp-2011-301706.
6. Kuwabara S, Misawa S, Kanai K, et al. Autologous peripheral blood stem cell transplantation for POEMS syndrome. Neurology. 2006;66(1):105–7.
7. D'Souza A, Hayman SR, Buadi F, et al. The utility of plasma vascular endothelial growth factor levels in the diagnosis and follow-up of patients with POEMS syndrome. Blood. 2011;118(17):4663–5. Prepublished on 02 Sept 2011 as doi:10.1182/blood-2011-06-362392.
8. Sekiguchi Y, Misawa S, Shibuya K, et al. Ambiguous effects of anti-VEGF monoclonal antibody (bevacizumab) for POEMS syndrome. Journal of Neurology, Neurosurgery, and Psychiatry. 2013;84(12):1346–8. Prepublished on 07 March 2013 as doi:10.1136/jnnp-2012-304874.
9. Soubrier M, Dubost JJ, Serre AF, et al. Growth factors in POEMS syndrome: evidence for a marked increase in circulating vascular endothelial growth factor. Arthritis Rheum. 1997;40(4):786–7.
10. Kanai K, Sawai S, Sogawa K, et al. Markedly upregulated serum interleukin-12 as a novel biomarker in POEMS syndrome. Neurology. 2012;79(6):575–82. Prepublished on 31 July 2012 as doi:10.1212/WNL. 0b013e318263c42b.
11. Yamada Y, Sawai S, Misawa S, et al. Multiple angiogenetic factors are upregulated in POEMS syndrome. Ann Hematol. 2013;92(2):245–8. Prepublished on 12 Oct 2012 as doi:10.1007/s00277-012-1583-2.
12. Wang C, Zhou YL, Cai H, et al. Markedly elevated serum total N-terminal propeptide of type I collagen is a novel marker for the diagnosis and follow up of patients with POEMS syndrome. Haematologica. 2014;99(6):e78–80. Prepublished on 25 March 2014 as doi:10.3324/haematol.2013.102962.
13. Naddaf E, Dispenzieri A, Mandrekar J, Mauermann ML. Thrombocytosis distinguishes POEMS syndrome from CIDP. Muscle & Nerve. 2015. Prepublished on 17 July 2015 as doi:10.1002/mus.24768.
14. Dispenzieri A. POEMS syndrome. Blood Rev. 2007;21(6):285–99.
15. Kelly JJ Jr, Kyle RA, Miles JM, Dyck PJ. Osteosclerotic myeloma and peripheral neuropathy. Neurology. 1983;33(2):202–10.
16. Koike H, Iijima M, Mori K, et al. Neuropathic pain correlates with myelinated fibre loss and cytokine profile in POEMS syndrome. J Neurol Neurosurg Psychiatry. 2008;79(10):1171–9.
17. Mauermann ML, Sorenson EJ, Dispenzieri A, Mandrekar J, Suarez GA, Dyck PJ. Uniform demyelination and more severe axonal loss distinguish POEMS syndrome from CIDP. J Neurol Neurosurg Psychiatry. 2012;83 (5):480–6. Prepublished on 08 March 2012 as doi:10.1136/jnnp-2011-301472.

18. Ghandi GY, Basu R, Dispenzieri A, Basu A, Montori V, Brennan MD. Endocrinopathy in POEMS syndrome: The Mayo Clinic experience. Mayo Clin Proc. 2007;82(7):836–42.

19. Dao LN, Hanson CA, Dispenzieri A, Morice WG, Kurtin PJ, Hoyer JD. Bone marrow histopathology in POEMS syndrome: a distinctive combination of plasma cell, lymphoid and myeloid findings in 87 patients. Blood. 2011;117(24):6438–6444. Prepublished on 10 March 2011 as doi:10.1182/blood-2010-11-316935.

20. Kaushik M, Pulido JS, Abreu R, Amselem L, Dispenzieri A. Ocular findings in patients with polyneuropathy, organomegaly, endocrinopathy, monoclonal gammopathy, and skin changes syndrome. Ophthalmology. 2011;118(4):778–82.

21. Cui R, Yu S, Huang X, Zhang J, Tian C, Pu C. Papilloedema is an independent prognostic factor for POEMS syndrome. Journal of Neurology. 2014;261(1):60–5. Prepublished on 22 Oct 2013 as doi:10. 1007/s00415-013-7143-4.

22. Cui RT, Yu SY, Huang XS, Zhang JT, Li F, Pu CQ. The characteristics of ascites in patients with POEMS syndrome. Annals of Hematology. 2013;92(12):1661–4. Prepublished on 03 July 2013 as doi:10.1007/ s00277-013-1829-7.

23. Dispenzieri A, Kyle RA, Lacy MQ, et al. POEMS syndrome: definitions and long-term outcome. Blood. 2003;101(7):2496–506.

24. Shi X, Hu S, Luo X, et al. CT characteristics in 24 patients with POEMS syndrome. Acta Radiologica. 2015. Prepublished on 13 Jan 2015 as doi:10. 1177/0284185114564614.

25. Glazebrook K, Guerra Bonilla FL, Johnson A, Leng S, Dispenzieri A. Computed tomography assessment of bone lesions in patients with POEMS syndrome. European radiology. 2015;25(2):497–504. Prepublished on 26 Nov 2014 as doi:10.1007/s00330-014-3428-y.

26. Li J, Zhou DB, Huang Z, et al. Clinical characteristics and long-term outcome of patients with POEMS syndrome in China. Annals of Hematology. 2011;90(7):819–826. Prepublished on 12 Jan 2011 as doi:10.1007/s00277-010-1149-0.

27. Lesprit P, Authier FJ, Gherardi R, et al. Acute arterial obliteration: a new feature of the POEMS syndrome? Medicine. 1996;75(4):226–32.

28. Dupont SA, Dispenzieri A, Mauermann ML, Rabinstein AA, Brown RD Jr. Cerebral infarction in POEMS syndrome: incidence, risk factors, and imaging characteristics. Neurology. 2009;73(16):1308–12.

29. Saida K, Kawakami H, Ohta M, Iwamura K. Coagulation and vascular abnormalities in Crow-Fukase syndrome. Muscle Nerve. 1997;20(4):486–92.

30. Watanabe O, Arimura K, Kitajima I, Osame M, Maruyama I. Greatly raised vascular endothelial growth factor (VEGF) in POEMS syndrome [letter]. Lancet. 1996;347(9002):702.

31. Watanabe O, Maruyama I, Arimura K, et al. Overproduction of vascular endothelial growth factor/vascular permeability factor is causative in Crow-Fukase (POEMS) syndrome. Muscle Nerve. 1998;21(11):1390–7.

32. Scarlato M, Previtali SC, Carpo M, et al. Polyneuropathy in POEMS syndrome: role of angiogenic factors in the pathogenesis. Brain. 2005;128 (Pt 8):1911–20.

33. Allam JS, Kennedy CC, Aksamit TR, Dispenzieri A. Pulmonary manifestations in patients with POEMS syndrome: a retrospective review of 137 patients. Chest. 2008;133(4):969–74.

34. Lesprit P, Godeau B, Authier FJ, et al. Pulmonary hypertension in POEMS syndrome: a new feature mediated by cytokines. Am J Respir Crit Care Med. 1998;157(3 Pt 1):907–11.

35. Li J, Tian Z, Zheng HY, et al. Pulmonary hypertension in POEMS syndrome. Haematologica. 2013;98(3):393–398. Prepublished on 18 Oct 2012 as doi:10.3324/haematol.2012.073031.

36. Stankowski-Drengler T, Gertz MA, Katzmann JA, et al. Serum immunoglobulin free light chain measurements and heavy chain isotype usage provide insight into disease biology in patients with POEMS syndrome. Am J Hematol. 2010;85(6):431–4.

37. Ye W, Wang C, Cai QQ, et al. Renal impairment in patients with polyneuropathy, organomegaly, endocrinopathy, monoclonal gammopathy and skin changes syndrome: incidence, treatment and outcome. Nephrology, Dialysis, Transplantation: Official Publication of the European Dialysis and Transplant Association—European Renal Association. 2015. Prepublished on 02 July 2015 as doi:10.1093/ndt/gfv261.

38. Soubrier MJ, Dubost JJ, Sauvezie BJ. POEMS syndrome: a study of 25 cases and a review of the literature. French Study Group on POEMS Syndrome. Am J Med. 1994;97(6):543–53.

39. Humeniuk MS, Gertz MA, Lacy MQ, et al. Outcomes of patients with POEMS syndrome treated initially with radiation. Blood. 2013;122(1):66–73. doi:10.1182/blood-2013-03-487025.

40. Li J, Zhang W, Jiao L, et al. Combination of melphalan and dexamethasone for patients with newly diagnosed POEMS syndrome. Blood. 2011;117(24):6445–9. Prepublished on 12 March 2011 as doi:10.1182/blood-2010-12-328112.

41. Jaccard A, Lazareth A, Karlin L, et al. A prospective Phase II trial of lenalidomide and dexamethasone (LEN-DEX) in POEMS syndrome. Blood. 2014;124(21).

42. Vannata B, Laurenti L, Chiusolo P, et al. Efficacy of lenalidomide plus dexamethasone for POEMS syndrome relapsed after autologous peripheral stem-cell transplantation. American Journal of Hematology. 2012;87 (6):641–2. Prepublished on 11 April 2012 as doi:10.1002/ajh.23195.

43. Dispenzieri A, Klein CJ, Mauermann ML. Lenalidomide therapy in a patient with POEMS syndrome. Blood. 2007;110(3):1075–6.

44. Royer B, Merlusca L, Abraham J, et al. Efficacy of lenalidomide in POEMS syndrome: a retrospective study of 20 patients. American Journal of Hematology. 2013;88(3):207–212. Prepublished on 22 Jan 2013 as doi:10.1002/ajh.23374.

45. Zagouri F, Kastritis E, Gavriatopoulou M, et al. Lenalidomide in patients with POEMS syndrome: a systematic review and pooled analysis. Leuk

Lymphoma. 2014;55(9):2018–2023. Prepublished on 04 Dec 2013 as doi:10.3109/10428194.2013.869329.

46. Kuwabara S, Misawa S, Kanai K, et al. Thalidomide reduces serum VEGF levels and improves peripheral neuropathy in POEMS syndrome. J Neurol Neurosurg Psychiatry. 2008;79(11):1255–7. Prepublished on 13 May 2008 as doi: 10.1136/jnnp.2008.150177 (jnnp.2008.150177 [pii]).

47. Katayama K, Misawa S, Sato Y, et al. Japanese POEMS syndrome with Thalidomide (J-POST) Trial: study protocol for a phase II/III multicentre, randomised, double-blind, placebo-controlled trial. BMJ Open. 2015;5(1): e007330. Prepublished on 13 Jan 2015 as doi:10.1136/bmjopen-2014-007330.

48. D'Souza A, Lacy M, Gertz M, et al. Long-term outcomes after autologous stem cell transplantation for patients with POEMS syndrome (osteosclerotic myeloma): a single-center experience. Blood. 2012;120 (1):56–62. Prepublished on 23 May 2012 as doi:10.1182/blood-2012-04-423178.

49. Karam C, Klein CJ, Dispenzieri A, et al. Polyneuropathy improvement following autologous stem cell transplantation for POEMS syndrome. Neurology. 2015;84(19):1981–7. Prepublished on 17 April 2015 as doi:10. 1212/WNL.0000000000001565.

50. Kojima H, Katsuoka Y, Katsura Y, et al. Successful treatment of a patient with POEMS syndrome by tandem high-dose chemotherapy with autologous CD34+ purged stem cell rescue. Int J Hematol. 2006;84 (2):182–5.

51. Dispenzieri A, Lacy MQ, Hayman SR, et al. Peripheral blood stem cell transplant for POEMS syndrome is associated with high rates of engraftment syndrome. Eur J Haematol. 2008;80(5):397–406.

52. Terracciano C, Fiore S, Doldo E, et al. Inverse correlation between VEGF and soluble VEGF receptor 2 in POEMS with AIDP responsive to intravenous immunoglobulin. Muscle Nerve. 2010;42(3):445–8.

53. Zhang L, Zhou YL, Zhang W, et al. Prevalence and risk factors for depression in newly diagnosed patients with POEMS syndrome. Leuk Lymphoma. 2014. Prepublished on 15 Feb 2014 as doi:10.3109/10428194. 2014.893309.

54. Kuwabara S, Misawa S, Kanai K, et al. Neurologic improvement after peripheral blood stem cell transplantation in POEMS syndrome. Neurology. 2008;71(21):1691–5.

55. Sethi S, Theis JD, Leung N, et al. Mass spectrometry-based proteomic diagnosis of renal immunoglobulin heavy chain amyloidosis. Clin J Am Soc Nephrol: CJASN. 2010;5(12):2180–7. Prepublished on 30 Oct 2010 as doi:10.2215/CJN.02890310.

56. Wang C, Su W, Zhang W, et al. Serum immunoglobulin free light chain and heavy/light chain measurements in POEMS syndrome. Ann Hematol. 2014;93(7):1201–6. Prepublished on 01 Feb 2014 as doi:10.1007/s00277-014-2019-y.

57. Dispenzieri A. Ushering in a new era for POEMS. Blood. 2011;117 (24):6405–6. Prepublished on 18 June 2011 as doi:10.1182/blood-2011-03-342675.

58. Castleman B, Iverson L, Menendez VP. Localized mediastinal lymph-node hyperplasia resembling thymoma. Cancer. 1956;9:822–30.
59. Fajgenbaum DC, van Rhee F, Nabel CS. HHV-8-negative, idiopathic multicentric Castleman disease: novel insights into biology, pathogenesis, and therapy. Blood. 2014;123(19):2924–2933. Prepublished on 14 March 2014 as doi:10.1182/blood-2013-12-545087.
60. Frizzera G, Banks PM, Massarelli G, Rosai J. A systemic lymphoproliferative disorder with morphologic features of Castleman's disease. Pathological findings in 15 patients. Am J Surg Pathol. 1983;7 (3):211–231.
61. Bowne WB, Lewis JJ, Filippa DA, et al. The management of unicentric and multicentric Castleman's disease: a report of 16 cases and a review of the literature. Cancer. 1999;85(3):706–17.
62. Chronowski GM, Ha CS, Wilder RB, Cabanillas F, Manning J, Cox JD. Treatment of unicentric and multicentric Castleman disease and the role of radiotherapy. Cancer. 2001;92(3):670–6.
63. Parez N, Bader-Meunier B, Roy CC, Dommergues JP. Paediatric Castleman disease: report of seven cases and review of the literature. Eur J Pediatr. 1999;158(8):631–7.
64. Soulier J, Grollet L, Oksenhendler E, et al. Kaposi's sarcoma-associated herpesvirus-like DNA sequences in multicentric Castleman's disease (see comment). Blood. 1995;86(4):1276–80.
65. Oksenhendler E, Duarte M, Soulier J, et al. Multicentric Castleman's disease in HIV infection: a clinical and pathological study of 20 patients. AIDS. 1996;10(1):61–7.
66. Keller AR, Hocholzer L, Castleman B. Hyaline-vascular and plasma-cell types of giant lymph node hyperplasia of the mediastinum and other locations. Cancer. 1972;29:670–83.
67. Chadburn A, Cesarman E, Nador RG, Liu YF, Knowles DM. Kaposi's sarcoma-associated herpesvirus sequences in benign lymphoid proliferations not associated with human immunodeficiency virus. Cancer. 1997;80(4):788–97.
68. Parravinci C, Corbellino M, Paulli M, et al. Expression of a virus-derived cytokine, KSHV vIL-6, in HIV-seronegative Castleman's disease. Am J Pathol. 1997;151(6):1517–22.
69. O'Leary J, Kennedy M, Howells D, et al. Cellular localisation of HHV-8 in Castleman's disease: is there a link with lymph node vascularity? Mol Pathol. 2000;53(2):69–76.
70. Suda T, Katano H, Delsol G, et al. HHV-8 infection status of AIDS-unrelated and AIDS-associated multicentric Castleman's disease. Pathol Int. 2001;51(9):671–9.
71. Rieu P, Noel LH, Droz D, et al. Glomerular involvement in lymphoproliferative disorders with hyperproduction of cytokines (Castleman, POEMS). Adv Nephrol Necker Hosp. 2000;30:305–31.
72. Brandt SJ, Bodine DM, Dunbar CE, Nienhuis AW. Retroviral-mediated transfer of interleukin-6 into hematopoietic cells of mice results in a syndrome resembling Castleman's disease. Curr Top Microbiol Immunol. 1990;166:37–41.

73. Menke DM, Tiemann M, Camoriano JK, et al. Diagnosis of Castleman's disease by identification of an immunophenotypically aberrant population of mantle zone B lymphocytes in paraffin-embedded lymph node biopsies. Am J Clin Pathol. 1996;105(3):268–76.
74. Nguyen DT, Diamond LW, Hansmann ML, et al. Castleman's disease. Differences in follicular dendritic network in the hyaline vascular and plasma cell variants. Histopathology. 1994;24(5):437–43.
75. Dispenzieri A. Castleman disease. Cancer Treat Res. 2008;142:293–330.
76. Oksenhendler E, Boulanger E, Galicier L, et al. High incidence of Kaposi sarcoma-associated herpesvirus-related non-Hodgkin lymphoma in patients with HIV infection and multicentric Castleman disease. Blood. 2002;99 (7):2331–6.
77. Loi S, Goldstein D, Clezy K, Milliken ST, Hoy J, Chipman M. Castleman's disease and HIV infection in Australia. HIV Med. 2004;5 (3):157–62.
78. Frizzera G, Peterson BA, Bayrd ED, Goldman A. A systemic lymphoproliferative disorder with morphologic features of Castleman's disease: clinical findings and clinicopathologic correlations in 15 patients. J Clin Oncol. 1985;3(9):1202–16.
79. Weisenburger DD. Membranous nephropathy. Its association with multicentric angiofollicular lymph node hyperplasia. Arch Pathol Lab Med. 1979;103(11):591–4.
80. Menke DM, Camoriano JK, Banks PM. Angiofollicular lymph node hyperplasia: a comparison of unicentric, multicentric, hyaline vascular, and plasma cell types of disease by morphometric and clinical analysis. Mod Pathol. 1992;5(5):525–30.
81. McCarty MJ, Vukelja SJ, Banks PM, Weiss RB. Angiofollicular lymph node hyperplasia (Castleman's disease). Cancer Treat Rev. 1995;21 (4):291–310.
82. Donaghy M, Hall P, Gawler J, et al. Peripheral neuropathy associated with Castleman's disease. J Neurol Sci. 1989;89:253–67.
83. Weisenburger DD, Nathwani BN, Winberg CD, Rappaport H. Multicentric angiofollicular lymph node hyperplasia: a clinicopathologic study of 16 cases. Hum Pathol. 1985;16(2):162–72.
84. Dispenzieri A, Armitage JO, Loe MJ, et al. The clinical spectrum of Castleman's disease. Am J Hematol. 2012;87(11):997–1002. Prepublished on 14 July 2012 as doi:10.1002/ajh.23291.
85. van Rhee F, Wong RS, Munshi N, et al. Siltuximab for multicentric Castleman's disease: a randomised, double-blind, placebo-controlled trial. Lancet Oncol. 2014;15(9):966–74. Prepublished on 22 July 2014 as doi:10.1016/S1470-2045(14)70319-5.
86. Nishimoto N, Kanakura Y, Aozasa K, et al. Humanized anti-interleukin-6 receptor antibody treatment of multicentric Castleman disease. Blood. 2005;106(8):2627–32.
87. Du MQ, Bacon CM, Isaacson PG. Kaposi sarcoma-associated herpesvirus/ human herpesvirus 8 and lymphoproliferative disorders. J Clin Pathol. 2007;60:1350–7

Chapter 4
Waldenstrom's Macroglobulinemia

Stephen M. Ansell, MD, PhD

Introduction

Waldenstrom's macroglobulinemia is an indolent B-cell malignancy defined by a lymphoplasmacytic infiltration in the bone marrow or in other organs including lymph nodes, liver, and spleen, as well as a monoclonal immunoglobulin M protein (IgM) in the serum [1, 2]. The infiltration of the bone marrow and extramedullary sites by malignant B lymphocytes, as well as elevated IgM levels, typically leads to symptoms associated with this disease. Patients may develop constitutional symptoms, pancytopenia, or organomegaly due to infiltration by malignant cells. They may also develop neuropathy, symptoms associated with immunoglobulin deposition or hyperviscosity due to the presence of increased serum levels of the monoclonal IgM protein [3, 4].

There is, however, significant heterogeneity in the clinical presentation of patients with this disease. Some patients may present with the symptoms listed above, but many patients are

S.M. Ansell, MD, PhD (✉)
Division of Hematology, Department of Medicine, Mayo Clinic,
200 First Street SW, Rochester, MN 55905, USA
e-mail: ansell.stephen@mayo.edu

© Springer Science+Business Media New York 2017
T.M. Zimmerman and S.K. Kumar (eds.),
Biology and Management of Unusual Plasma Cell Dyscrasias,
DOI 10.1007/978-1-4419-6848-7_4

asymptomatic at the time the diagnosis is made. Some of these asymptomatic patients have very low serum IgM levels, a modest increase in lymphoplasmacytic cells in the bone marrow and no evidence of anemia or organomegaly. Many of the asymptomatic patients have a very indolent disease course, and some do not develop overt disease. Based on the extent of infiltration in the bone marrow and the serum IgM levels, asymptomatic patients can be further categorized as having a monoclonal gammopathy of undetermined significance (MGUS) or smoldering Waldenstrom's macroglobulinemia.

While Waldenstrom's macroglobulinemia typically follows an indolent course, the disease remains incurable with current therapy and the median survival for symptomatic patients is approximately 8 years [5]. Furthermore, many patients are diagnosed with Waldenstrom's macroglobulinemia at an advanced age and approximately half of the patients die from causes unrelated to the disease. Therefore, due to the incurable nature of the disease, the heterogeneous clinical presentation, as well as the presence of multiple comorbidities and competing causes of death, the decision to treat patients as well as the choice of treatment can be complex. A number of consensus meetings involving experts in the field have outlined recommended treatment approaches [6–8]. Despite this, the treating physician may still be faced with a difficult treatment decision in a complex patient with an uncommon disease.

Epidemiology

The incidence of Waldenstrom's macroglobulinemia is approximately 5 cases per million persons per year, and Waldenstrom's macroglobulinemia accounts for approximately 1–2 % of all hematological cancers [9, 10]. The incidence of this disease is highest among Caucasians, but is rare in other population groups [11]. The majority of new patients are male, and the median age at diagnosis varies between 63 and 68 years [3]. Patients with a previously diagnosed MGUS are at increased risk for progression to Waldenstrom's macroglobulinemia [12]. In population-based studies of individuals with MGUS, the rate of progression from

IgM-MGUS to Waldenstrom's macroglobulinemia has been noted to be approximately 1.5–2 % per year [13–15].

While the development of Waldenstrom's macroglobulinemia is generally thought to be sporadic, there are studies suggesting a familial predisposition for the disease [16–18]. Familial clustering of Waldenstrom's macroglobulinemia, as well as a significant increase in the frequency of IgM-MGUS in first-degree relatives of Waldenström patients, is strongly suggestive of familial risk [17]. Based on the assumption that Waldenstrom's macroglobulinemia and IgM-MGUS may share common susceptibility genes, strong linkages have been identified involving chromosomes 1q, 3q, and 4q [13]. Furthermore, several studies have suggested a familial association between MGUS/Waldenstrom's macroglobulinemia and chronic antigenic stimulation [18–21]. It was recently shown that a sizable minority of patients with IgM-MGUS/Waldenstrom's macroglobulinemia reacted with a protein of unknown function called paratarg-7 (P-7) [22]. Relatives of patients with IgM-MGUS/Waldenstrom's macroglobulinemia analyzed using an anti-P-7-paraprotein showed that the hyperphosphorylated state of this protein (pP7) is inherited as a dominant trait. It was also shown that carriers of pP7 have a substantially increased risk of developing IgM-MGUS/Waldenstrom's macroglobulinemia [22]. Hyperphosphorylated P-7 is therefore the first biological entity that provides a potential explanation for the familial clustering of cases of IgM-MGUS/Waldenstrom's macroglobulinemia.

Diagnosis

In recent years, efforts to more clearly define Waldenstrom's macroglobulinemia have been made by the World Health Organization (WHO) Lymphoma Classification [23], the consensus group formed at the Second International Workshop on Waldenstrom's Macroglobulinemia [1], and the Mayo Clinic [24]. However, the diagnostic criteria for Waldenstrom's macroglobulinemia by these respective groups are not identical. All groups recognize Waldenstrom's macroglobulinemia as a lymphoplasmacytic lymphoma associated with an IgM monoclonal protein in the serum. The WHO definition, however, includes lymphomas other than lymphoplasmacytic lymphoma and does not restrict the monoclonal protein to IgM but also allows IgG or IgA. In contrast, the Second International Workshop on Waldenström's Macroglobulinemia restricts the diagnosis of Waldenstrom's macroglobulinemia exclusively to cases with lymphoplasmacytic lymphoma and an IgM monoclonal protein. The Second International Workshop on Waldenström's Macroglobulinemia also removed the requirement for a minimum degree of bone marrow involvement or a threshold serum level of IgM to fulfill the diagnosis, but instead allowed for any detectable amount of either. In contrast, Mayo Clinic criteria require at least 10 % involvement of the bone marrow by lymphoplasmacytic lymphoma in asymptomatic patients. As regards the analysis of pathologic features, the WHO criteria focus predominantly on nodal involvement, whereas studies at Mayo Clinic suggest that the analysis of most cases of Waldenstrom's macroglobulinemia should be bone marrow based.

Lymphoplasmacytic lymphoma, whether involving the bone marrow or nodal sites, typically exhibits a cytologic spectrum ranging from small lymphocytes with clumped chromatin, inconspicuous nucleoli, and sparse cytoplasm to well-formed plasma cells [1, 25]. Also commonly present are "plasmacytoid lymphocytes," which have cytologic features of both lymphocytes and plasma cells, although the cytology and extent of plasmacytic differentiation may vary from case to case. Involvement of lymph nodes is typically characterized by paracortical and hilar infiltration with frequent sparing of the subscapular and marginal sinuses. The bone marrow involvement usually exhibits a combination of nodular, paratrabecular, and interstitial infiltration. Plasma cells containing Dutcher bodies are commonly present.

The lymphoplasmacytic cells present in Waldenstrom's macroglobulinemia display a broad cytologic spectrum and the immunophenotypic features of the lymphocytic and plasmacytic components can be rather varied. The lymphocytic infiltrate commonly displays high levels of surface CD19, CD20, and immunoglobulin light-chain expression, but the malignant B lymphocytes typically lack CD10 expression [25]. In approximately half of the cases, malignant lymphocytes show some degree of CD5 expression; however, the intensity of expression is not as strong as on malignant B cells from patients with chronic lymphocytic leukemia/small lymphocytic lymphoma or mantle cell lymphoma. The plasmacytic component expresses the same immunoglobulin light chain as the lymphocytic component, is positive for CD138 and shows diminished expression of B-cell-associated antigens such as CD19, CD20, and PAX5. Overall, the lymphoplasmacytic lymphoma cells are positive for surface IgM, and on the basis of the WHO criteria, they may express any immunoglobulin isotype. In cases that have undergone isotype switching, the phenotype of the plasma cells closely resembles that of myeloma plasma cells with strong CD38 and CD138 co-expression and complete lack of CD19 expression. Waldenstrom's macroglobulinemia tumor cells have also been shown to variably express CD25, CD27, FMC7, and Bcl2, and lack expression of Bcl6 and CD75.

Conventional cytogenetic analyses initially determined deletions of chromosome 6q to be the most common recurrent abnormality in Waldenstrom macroglobulinemia, and this abnormality was identified in approximately half of the patients studied [26]. In a study by Schop et al. [27], 23 % of patients with an abnormal karyotype had a 6q deletion, while FISH analysis found deletions of 6q in 42 % of patients. Further analysis to assess minimal areas of deletion used multiple FISH probes on the 6q arm, and the results suggested a minimal deleted region at 6q23–24.3 [28]. Although the deletion of 6q is present in around 50 % of Waldenstrom macroglobulinemia patients, its presence cannot be used for diagnosis of the disease as the deletion is widely observed in other B-cell malignancies, such as marginal zone lymphoma, multiple myeloma and chronic lymphocytic leukemia [29–32].

Recent data obtained from whole-genome sequencing of Waldenstrom's macroglobulinemia patients reported a mutation in *MYD88* in 90 % of cases (46/51), which leads to a leucine-to-proline substitution in codon 265 (L265P) [33]. This *MYD88* mutation is likely to become a biomarker for differentiating Waldenstrom's macroglobulinemia from other related entities such as marginal zone lymphoma, where *MYD88* L265P was detected in less than 10 % of cases. Furthermore, a low prevalence of *MYD88* mutations in IgM-MGUS suggests that the mutation is associated with disease progression or that there is more than one type of IgM-MGUS, with only certain types of IgM-MGUS progressing to Waldenstrom's macroglobulinemia.

Gene expression profile (GEP) analysis of Waldenstrom's macroglobulinemia has also provided useful information about the transcriptional signature of the disease. Two studies have studied the similarities and differences in GEP between Waldenstrom's macroglobulinemia, chronic lymphocytic lymphoma (CLL), multiple myeloma, normal B cells, and normal plasma cells [34, 35]. These studies have identified similarities between GEP in Waldenstrom's macroglobulinemia and CLL. When analyzed in an unsupervised fashion, gene expression in Waldenstrom's macroglobulinemia cells clustered with CLL rather than with multiple myeloma [34]. This may not be surprising as both Waldenstrom's macroglobulinemia and CLL have a strong B-cell signature, are characterized by expression of similar B-cell markers and are defined by low proliferation rates and a lack of immunoglobulin heavy-chain mutations [35]. The GEP of Waldenstrom's macroglobulinemia and CLL shared similar profiles, particularly with regard to cell surface markers and cytokines such as IL-10 [34, 35].

A significant finding in both studies was the high level of IL-6 transcript expression in Waldenstrom's macroglobulinemia when compared to multiple myeloma, CLL, and normal B cells [34, 35]. IL-6 is an inflammatory cytokine that increases lymphocyte activity, including antibody production [36]. IL-6 plays a key role by activating the MAPK pathway, and while the genetic studies found no specific mutations in *MAPK*, its activity was notably increased, likely due to the upregulation of IL-6 [34]. The increase in IL-6 expression in Waldenstrom's macroglobulinemia cells, more so than in normal B cells, is suggestive of an autocrine loop. IL-6 binds to the tyrosine kinase receptor Janus kinases (JAK) 1 and 2, which activate the downstream transcription factor Stat3, leading to increases in gene transcription and IgM production [37]. Recently, a functional relationship between IL-6, RANTES (CCL5), and IgM secretion was observed and appears to be mediated through the JAK/STAT and PI3K pathways [38]. Although the specific mechanisms of increased immunoglobulin secretion in Waldenstrom's macroglobulinemia are still not entirely understood, the pathogenic role of IL-6 and the JAK/STAT pathway in Waldenstrom's macroglobulinemia merits further study.

Clinical Presentation

Infiltration of the bone marrow by malignant cells and the increased levels of circulating IgM protein in patients with Waldenstrom's macroglobulinemia are responsible for the majority of the signs and symptoms associated with this malignancy. While some patients with Waldenstrom's macroglobulinemia are asymptomatic at diagnosis, others present with anemia, bleeding, or neurological complaints [39]. Additionally, because IgM protein circulates in the serum as a large pentameric molecule, many patients present with symptoms associated with immunoglobulin deposition and hyperviscosity syndrome [40]. Symptoms due to hyperviscosity syndrome have been reported in approximately one-third of Waldenstrom's macroglobulinemia patients and include skin and mucosal bleeding, retinopathy, other visual disturbances, and cold sensitivity [39, 41].

Due to an absence of curative therapies, as well as significant variability in clinical presentation and comorbidities, when and how to treat patients diagnosed with Waldenstrom's macroglobulinemia can be a challenging decision. Before treatment can even be considered, it is important to differentiate between Waldenstrom's macroglobulinemia, IgM-MGUS and smoldering Waldenstrom's macroglobulinemia, as the appropriate treatment strategy varies depending on the diagnosis. To aid in this decision-making process, Mayo Clinic has described diagnostic criteria to differentiate between these IgM gammopathies based on the extent of bone marrow involvement and the presence or absence of symptomatic disease (see Table 4.1) [24].

Prognostic Factors

After the diagnosis of Waldenstrom's macroglobulinemia is made, the next step is to use a risk-adapted approach to determine how best to manage the disease. The International Prognostic Staging System for Waldenstrom Macroglobulinemia (IPSSWM), a multicenter collaborative project, used five adverse prognostic factors to define three different risk groups for patients with Waldenstrom's macroglobulinemia [42]. These factors include age >65 years,

Table 4.1 Diagnostic criteria for Waldenstrom's macroglobulinemia [24]

Waldenstrom's macroglobulinemia	IgM monoclonal gammopathy (regardless of the size of the M protein) with >10 % bone marrow lymphoplasmacytic infiltration (usually intertrabecular) by small lymphocytes that exhibit plasmacytoid or plasma cell differentiation and a typical immunophenotype (surface IgM$^+$, CD5$^-$, CD10$^-$, CD19$^+$, CD20$^+$, CD23$^-$) that satisfactorily excludes other lymphoproliferative disorders including chronic lymphocytic leukemia and mantle cell lymphoma
IgM-MGUS	Serum IgM monoclonal protein level <3 g/dL, bone marrow lymphoplasmacytic infiltration <10 %, and no evidence of anemia, constitutional symptoms, hyperviscosity, lymphadenopathy, or hepatosplenomegaly
Smoldering Waldenstrom's macroglobulinemia (also referred to as indolent or asymptomatic Waldenstrom's macroglobulinemia)	Serum IgM monoclonal protein level ≥3 g/dL and/or bone marrow lymphoplasmacytic infiltration ≥10 %, and no evidence of end-organ damage, such as anemia, constitutional symptoms, hyperviscosity, lymphadenopathy, or hepatosplenomegaly that can be attributed to a lymphoplasmacytic disorder

hemoglobin <11.5 g/dL, platelet count <100,000/mcL, β_2-microglobulin >3 mg/L, and monoclonal IgM protein >7 g/dL. Patients with 0–1, 2, or >2 of these factors are considered to be at low risk, intermediate risk, or high risk, with 5-year survival rates of 87, 68, and 37 % respectively. While the IPSSWM is not specifically used to determine the most appropriate treatment regimen, understanding a patient's risk group may be helpful in deciding whether and when treatment is necessary. Conversely, many asymptomatic patients may not require any therapy at all. To illustrate this point, a study by Garcia-Sanz et al. found that 50 % of patients who were asymptomatic at diagnosis did not require therapy for almost 3 years [39]. Similarly, one in ten patients who were initially observed without therapy did not require therapy for ten years. These data highlight the need to carefully consider a patient's prognostic risk prior to starting treatment so as to limit therapy to only those patients in whom it is necessary.

Indications for Treatment

To better identify the patients with Waldenstrom's macroglobulinemia who should receive therapy, a consensus panel at the Second International Workshop on Waldenstrom Macroglobulinemia agreed that treatment should be initiated in patients with a specific set of clinical findings and/or laboratory parameters [43]. Specifically, it was recommended that treatment be initiated in patients presenting with any of the following: constitutional symptoms including fever, night sweats or weight loss; lymphadenopathy or splenomegaly; hemoglobin <10 g/dL or a platelet count lower than 100×10^9/L due to bone marrow infiltration; as well as complications of Waldenstrom's macroglobulinemia including symptomatic sensorimotor peripheral neuropathy, systemic amyloidosis, renal insufficiency, or symptomatic cryoglobulinemia. It was also recommended that patients with IgM-MGUS and smoldering (asymptomatic) Waldenstrom's macroglobulinemia with preserved hematological function should be observed without treatment. Furthermore, all patients should be evaluated for symptoms of hyperviscosity (rarely observed with IgM levels <4 g/dL) such as visual deterioration, neurological symptoms, or unexplained bleeding. These patients should undergo plasmapheresis if necessary prior to receiving chemotherapy or a monoclonal antibody such as rituximab [44].

Initial Therapy

Initial therapy for previously untreated patients with symptomatic Waldenstrom's macroglobulinemia may involve various chemotherapeutic combinations typically with the addition of the

CD20⁺-directed antibody, rituximab [45]. However, low-risk patients with symptomatic Waldenstrom's macroglobulinemia may sometimes receive rituximab alone as first-line treatment. Treatment regimens containing nucleoside analogs, such as fludarabine, have demonstrated good efficacy in symptomatic Waldenstrom's macroglobulinemia patients particularly when used in combination, including fludarabine/cyclophosphamide/rituximab (FCR) and fludarabine/rituximab (FR). In a multicenter prospective study of previously untreated patients with symptomatic disease, the FCR regimen was associated with an overall response rate of 79 %, including 12 % who had a complete remission and 21 % who had very good partial remissions [46]. Significant myelosuppression, however, is a limitation of this combination, as grade 3 or 4 neutropenia was reported in 45 % of treatment courses and was the main reason for discontinuing treatment. A separate study similarly examined patients who received six cycles of fludarabine combined with eight infusions of rituximab (FR) [47]. Of the 43 patients enrolled, complete responses were achieved in two patients, with 81 % of patients achieving either a very good partial response or partial response. Similar toxicities to the FCR regimen were seen, and neutropenia, thrombocytopenia, and pneumonia of grade 3 or higher were reported in 63 % of patients treated with FR.

Despite the clinical activity of nucleoside analog-based therapies in the treatment of Waldenstrom's macroglobulinemia, an increased incidence of transformation to large cell lymphoma, as well as the development of myelodysplasia, has been associated with the use of these agents. A recent study followed 439 patients with Waldenstrom's macroglobulinemia, of whom 193 were previously treated with nucleoside analogs, 136 who were treated without a nucleoside analog, and 110 who were observed without treatment. All were followed for a median of five years [48]. Among the nucleoside analog-treated cohort, 5 % of patients transformed and 2 % developed myelodysplasia, whereas only one patient transformed within the other groups. These data suggest that while nucleoside analog-based therapeutic regimens are effective, the additional long-term risks associated with these therapies must be taken into account when deciding upon an initial treatment strategy for patients with Waldenstrom's macroglobulinemia.

Initially considered to be the standard of care, alkylating agents have also been used in patients with Waldenstrom's macroglobulinemia. Over time, combinations of alkylating agents, such as chlorambucil and cyclophosphamide, have been studied with vinca alkaloids, nucleoside analogs, and anthracyclines and have been shown to be effective [49–52]. The addition of rituximab to alkylator-based combinations has further increased patient response rates. In a prospective, randomized trial including patients with Waldenstrom's macroglobulinemia treated with R-CHOP or CHOP without rituximab, a significantly higher overall response rate was achieved in the patient group receiving chemoimmunotherapy as compared to chemotherapy alone (94 % vs. 67 %, $p = 0.008$), with no major differences noted in toxicity [53]. Furthermore, patients in the R-CHOP group experienced a significantly longer time to treatment failure as compared to patients in the CHOP arm (63 months vs. 22 months, $p = 0.003$). Similarly, significant activity with less toxicity has been achieved in Waldenstrom macroglobulinemia patients with other combinations containing alkylating agents and rituximab, suggesting that such regimens may be preferable as initial therapy for this disease [44]. For example, treatment with dexamethasone, rituximab, and cyclophosphamide (DRC) yielded an overall response rate of 83 % in previously untreated patients, 7 % of whom had a complete response to therapy [54]. Toxicity was mild, and only 9 % of patients experienced grade 3 or 4 neutropenia.

Bendamustine, a newer alkylating agent, has also shown significant activity in Waldenstrom macroglobulinemia, particularly when combined with rituximab. In a cohort of relapsed and refractory patients treated with bendamustine in combination with rituximab, an overall response rate of 83 % was seen [55]. While the therapy was well tolerated, there was an increased incidence of myelosuppression in patients who had previously been treated with nucleoside analogs [48]. Bendamustine plus rituximab has now become a standard frontline therapy in Waldenstrom macroglobulinemia based on a randomized comparison with R-CHOP [56]. When compared with R-CHOP, treatment with bendamustine plus rituximab resulted in fewer relapses, was better tolerated and was associated with a longer progression-free survival, despite identical response rates for both regimens.

Rapid and durable patient responses have also been achieved with the proteasome inhibitor bortezomib when used in combination with rituximab in this disease. When bortezomib, dexamethasone, and rituximab (BDR) were administered to previously untreated, but symptomatic Waldenstrom's macroglobulinemia patients, the overall response rate was extremely high (96 %) and responses occurred at a median of 1.4 months [57]. Unfortunately, a high incidence of peripheral neuropathy led to the discontinuation of bortezomib in almost two-thirds of patients. Similar results were seen in a separate study that reported an overall response rate of 88 % in patients with symptomatic Waldenstrom's macroglobulinemia who received only bortezomib and rituximab [58]. In this study, no grade 3 or 4 neuropathies were reported, and the most significant adverse event was neutropenia in 12 % of patients.

When used as a single-agent, rituximab has been associated with response rates ranging from 29 to 65 %, and single-agent rituximab is a reasonable option in the treatment of Waldenstrom's macroglobulinemia. This approach may be most appropriate in low-risk patients with symptomatic disease and minimal hematological compromise, as well as in patients with IgM-related neuropathy requiring treatment [44]. In a study of 69 symptomatic patients, an overall response rate of 52 % was reported following administration of rituximab as a single agent [59]. When using rituximab as a single agent, clinicians need to be aware of the paradoxical increase in IgM protein levels seen in some patients, known as the rituximab "flare" [44, 60]. IgM levels may remain elevated for up to 4 months following treatment with rituximab, and while this does not necessarily indicate treatment failure, additional treatment such as plasmapheresis may be necessary to alleviate symptoms of hyperviscosity.

Based on the variety of different agents that are clinically active in this disease, a risk-adapted approach to the management of Waldenstrom's macroglobulinemia is necessary. Three groups of patients have previously been identified [44]. Firstly, patients with IgM-MGUS or smoldering (asymptomatic) Waldenstrom's macroglobulinemia and normal hematological function constitute a low-risk group. Second, symptomatic Waldenstrom's macroglobulinemia patients with modest hematological compromise, IgM-related neuropathy or hemolytic anemia are at intermediate risk of disease progression and subsequent morbidity or mortality.

Thirdly, Waldenstrom's macroglobulinemia patients who have constitutional symptoms, significant hematological compromise, bulky disease or hyperviscosity have a high risk of disease progression and early mortality. Utilizing these risk groups, we recommend the following: (1) Patients with IgM-MGUS or smoldering (asymptomatic) Waldenstrom macroglobulinemia and preserved hematological function should be observed without initial therapy. (2) Symptomatic Waldenstrom's macroglobulinemia patients with modest hematological compromise, IgM-related neuropathy, or hemolytic anemia unresponsive to corticosteroids should receive four standard doses of rituximab alone without maintenance therapy. (3) Waldenstrom's macroglobulinemia patients who have significant constitutional symptoms, profound hematological compromise, bulky disease, or hyperviscosity should be treated with chemoimmunotherapy using either bendamustine in combination with rituximab or the DRC regimen (dexamethasone, rituximab, and cyclophosphamide). Any patient with symptoms of hyperviscosity should first be treated with plasmapheresis (see mSMART algorithm in Fig. 4.1) [44].

Management of Relapsed Disease

Even though there are high overall response rates associated with the upfront treatment regimens and despite the introduction of new therapeutic agents into initial treatment combinations, studies have not clearly demonstrated a significant improvement in the overall outcome of patients with Waldenstrom's macroglobulinemia treated during the last 25 years [61]. These findings highlight the need for more effective agents to further improve patient survival, especially in patients who have failed previous treatment regimens. Fortunately, new therapies and new treatment combinations are currently being tested in patients with refractory and relapsed disease.

Examples of new agents being used in patients with relapsed disease include immunomodulating drugs (IMiDs), including thalidomide and lenalidomide, which have been studied in Waldenstrom's macroglobulinemia in combination with rituximab as these agents enhance rituximab-mediated antibody-dependent

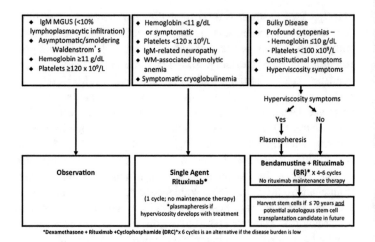

| IgM MGUS (<10% lymphoplasmacytic infiltration) • Asymptomatic/smoldering Waldenstrom's • Hemoglobin ≥11 g/dL • Platelets ≥120 x 10⁹/L | • Hemoglobin <11 g/dL or symptomatic • Platelets <120 x 10⁹/L • IgM-related neuropathy • WM-associated hemolytic anemia • Symptomatic cryoglobulinemia | • Bulky Disease • Profound cytopenias – - Hemoglobin ≤10 g/dL - Platelets <100 x10⁹/L • Constitutional symptoms • Hyperviscosity symptoms |

Hyperviscosity symptoms

Yes   No

Plasmapheresis

| Observation | Single Agent Rituximab* (1 cycle; no maintenance therapy) *plasmapheresis if hyperviscosity develops with treatment | Bendamustine + Rituximab (BR)* x 4-6 cycles No rituximab maintenance therapy

Harvest stem cells if ≤ 70 years and potential autologous stem cell transplantation candidate in future |

*Dexamethasone + Rituximab +Cyclophosphamide (DRC)*x 6 cycles is an alternative if the disease burden is low

Fig. 4.1 Mayo clinic [mayo stratification of macroglobulinemia and risk-adapted therapy (mSMART)] consensus for management of newly diagnosed Waldenstrom's macroglobulinemia [44]. *MGUS* monoclonal gammopathy of undetermined significance. SI conversion factor: to convert hemoglobin values to g/L, multiply by 10

cellular cytotoxicity (ADCC) [62]. However, despite relatively high overall response rates, treatment with both thalidomide and lenalidomide has been associated with significant toxicity [63]. In the case of lenalidomide and rituximab, the clinical trial was closed early due to reports of significant anemia, which occurred in 13 of 16 treated patients [64]. Therefore, while these agents have demonstrated significant clinical activity, further studies are necessary to identify the optimal dose and schedule of the drug that results in maximal activity with minimal toxicity.

Everolimus, a mammalian target of rapamycin (mTOR) inhibitor, has also been studied in patients with Waldenstrom's macroglobulinemia, due to the previously described role of the PI3K/Akt/mTOR signal transduction pathway as a driver of tumor viability in various hematological diseases, including Waldenstrom's macroglobulinemia [65]. When everolimus was used as a single agent in patients with relapsed or refractory Waldenstrom's macroglobulinemia, an overall response rate of 70 % was reported with a 12-month progression-free survival of 62 % [66]. The drug did have significant toxicity with 56 % of patients developing grade 3 or greater toxicities that required dose reductions in more than half of the patients. However, despite its toxicity profile, single-agent everolimus appears to be a potential new therapeutic option for the treatment of Waldenstrom's macroglobulinemia.

Due to antitumor activity seen in preclinical studies of the histone deacetylase inhibitor panobinostat in Waldenstrom's macroglobulinemia cell lines, this agent has been studied in a phase II trial of patients with refractory or relapsed disease [67]. Panobinostat was found to be an active in this patient population with an overall response rate of 60 %. Because of frequent hematological toxicities, the dose of panobinostat was decreased from 30 mg three times per week to 25 mg three times per week, and the lower dosing schedule was better tolerated.

In addition to chemotherapeutics, other novel antibodies targeting CD20 are also in development in Waldenstrom's macroglobulinemia to improve upon the response rates seen with single-agent rituximab and to limit the "flare" in IgM often seen with rituximab therapy. One such monoclonal antibody is ofatumumab that targets a different epitope on CD20. Ofatumumab targets an epitope encompassing both the large and small extracellular loops of CD20, whereas rituximab targets only the large loop [68]. Ofatumumab has been studied as a single agent in 37 patients with Waldenstrom's macroglobulinemia, 28 of whom had received a median of three prior therapies [69]. An overall response rate of 59 % was reported, and there was a lower incidence of IgM "flare" as compared to what is typically seen with rituximab. The toxicity profile, which included the development of infection in 15 patients, was deemed to be acceptable, making ofatumumab a further therapeutic option in Waldenstrom's macroglobulinemia, particularly in patients with refractory disease.

Whole-genome sequencing of tumor cells in Waldenstrom's macroglobulinemia has revealed a highly prevalent somatic mutation in *MYD88* [33]. *MYD88* L265P is present in >90 % of patients with Waldenstrom's macroglobulinemia, and supports malignant growth via signaling involving Bruton's tyrosine kinase (BTK). Ibrutinib, an inhibitor of BTK signaling, induces apoptosis of malignant cells bearing *MYD88* L265P. In a clinical trial of ibrutinib in relapsed or refractory patients with Waldenstrom's macroglobulinemia [70], the overall response rate including minor responses or better was 90.5 %, with a major response rate (partial response or better) of 73 % and a median time to response of 4 weeks. Rapid reductions in serum IgM and improvement in hematocrit occurred in most patients receiving ibrutinib, and the estimated 2-year progression-free survival was 69 %. Furthermore, response rates were higher in patients with mutated *MYD88* compared to wild type. The study confirmed that ibrutinib is highly active and well tolerated in patients with relapsed or refractory Waldenstrom's macroglobulinemia and this agent is now an approved therapy in this disease. It is typically used as the standard second-line agent in relapsed patients.

Finally, stem cell transplantation (SCT) is another potential option in the treatment of patients with advanced Waldenstrom's macroglobulinemia. Autologous SCT is relatively well tolerated, and durable complete responses have been reported [44]. In a retrospective analysis of 158 heavily pretreated patients with Waldenstrom's macroglobulinemia who underwent autologous (SCT), nearly half of the patients remained in remission at 5 years, with a non-relapse mortality rate of only 3.8 %. Five-year progression-free survival and overall survival rates were 40 and 68 %, respectively [71]. While additional prospective studies are needed, these initial results suggest that autologous SCT may have a place in the treatment of Waldenstrom's macroglobulinemia, particularly in younger patients.

A similar retrospective study has also been performed to assess the role of allogeneic SCT in the treatment of Waldenstrom's macroglobulinemia. In a review of 86 patients with Waldenstrom's macroglobulinemia who received an allograft after either myeloablative or reduced-intensity conditioning (RIC) regimens, both the myeloablative and RIC regimens were associated with significantly higher risks of non-relapse mortality at 3 years (33 and 23 %, respectively) [72]. At present, allogeneic SCT is not considered a routine therapeutic option for patients with Waldenstrom's macroglobulinemia outside of a clinical trial.

As there is currently no standard approach to the management of patients with relapsed Waldenstrom's macroglobulinemia, the approach of our group (Fig. 4.2) is to consider all patients for participation in a clinical trial either as definitive therapy for their disease or as preparative therapy prior to considering an autologous SCT [44]. For patients who are ineligible or unwilling to go on a

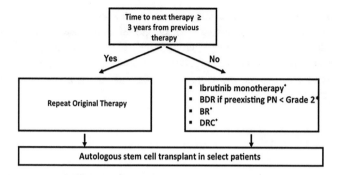

*If not previously used.
For multiply relapsed or refractory disease, in addition to the regimens listed above, consider nucleoside analog (cladribine or fludarabine)-based regimens or everolimus as alternatives.
DRC = Dexamethasone + Rituximab + Cyclophosphamide; BR = Bendamustine + Rituximab; BDR = Bortezomib (weekly), Dexamethasone + Rituximab; PN= peripheral neuropathy

Fig. 4.2 Mayo clinic [mayo stratification of macroglobulinemia and risk-adapted therapy (mSMART)] consensus for management of relapsed Waldenstrom's macroglobulinemia [44]

clinical trial, the choice of therapy is determined by their response to frontline treatment. Because responses to initial therapies are often delayed and can occur a year or more after initiating treatment, we recommend using a 3-year cutoff to determine treatment. For patients with a durable response that lasted >3 years, the original therapy can be repeated. For patients who have an inadequate response to initial therapy or a response lasting <3 years, an alternative approach should be used. Our group will commonly use ibrutinib in these patients if not previously used. An autologous stem cell transplant can also be considered in eligible patients with relapsed disease.

Conclusions

Waldenstrom's macroglobulinemia is a rare disease, and practicing physicians may infrequently treat these patients. Patients may present with a variety of clinical findings, and many patients do not require treatment initially. When patients do require therapy, it is important to select therapies that do not limit future treatment options. To provide a simple risk-adapted approach to managing patients with Waldenstrom's macroglobulinemia, we have outlined what we feel to be a rational approach to this disease [44]. These recommendations are regularly updated as new data become available and the most current guidelines are available at www. mSMART.org.

References

1. Owen RG, Treon SP, Al-Katib A, et al. Clinicopathological definition of Waldenstrom's macroglobulinemia: consensus panel recommendations from the second international workshop on Waldenstrom's macroglobulinemia. Semin Oncol. 2003;30:110–5.
2. Dimopoulos MA, Kyle RA, Anagnostopoulos A, Treon SP. Diagnosis and management of Waldenstrom's macroglobulinemia. J Clin Oncol. 2005;23:1564–77.
3. Dimopoulos MA, Panayiotidis P, Moulopoulos LA, Sfikakis P, Dalakas M. Waldenstrom's macroglobulinemia: clinical features, complications, and management. J Clin Oncol. 2000;18:214–26.
4. Vijay A, Gertz MA. Waldenstrom macroglobulinemia. Blood. 2007;109:5096–103.
5. Kastritis E, Kyrtsonis MC, Hatjiharissi E, et al. No significant improvement in the outcome of patients with Waldenström's macroglobulinemia treated over the last 25 years. Am J Hematol. 2011;86(6):479–83.
6. Gertz MA, Anagnostopoulos A, Anderson K, et al. Treatment recommendations in Waldenstrom's macroglobulinemia: consensus panel recommendations from the second international workshop on Waldenstrom's macroglobulinemia. Semin Oncol. 2003;30:121–6.
7. Treon SP, Gertz MA, Dimopoulos M, et al. Update on treatment recommendations from the third international workshop on Waldenstrom's macroglobulinemia. Blood. 2006;107:3442–6.
8. Dimopoulos MA, Gertz MA, Kastritis E, et al. Update on treatment recommendations from the fourth international workshop on Waldenstrom's macroglobulinemia. J Clin Oncol. 2009;27:120–6.
9. Herrinton LJ, Weiss NS. Incidence of Waldenstrom's macroglobulinemia. Blood. 1993;82:3148–50.
10. Groves FD, Travis LB, Devesa SS, Ries LA, Fraumeni JF Jr. Waldenstrom's macroglobulinemia: incidence patterns in the United States, 1988–1994. Cancer. 1998;82:1078–81.
11. Benjamin M, Reddy S, Brawley OW. Myeloma and race: a review of the literature. Cancer Metastasis Rev. 2003;22:87–93.
12. Kyle RA, Therneau TM, Rajkumar SV, et al. A long-term study of prognosis in monoclonal gammopathy of undetermined significance. N Engl J Med. 2002;346(8):564–9.

13. McMaster ML, Goldin LR, Bai Y, et al. Genome wide linkage screen for Waldenstrom macroglobulinemia susceptibility loci in high-risk families. Am J Hum Genet. 2006;79(4):695–701.

14. Kyle RA, Therneau TM, Rajkumar SV, et al. Long-term follow-up of IgM monoclonal gammopathy of undetermined significance. Blood. 2003;102 (10):3759–64.

15. Kyle RA, Therneau TM, Rajkumar SV, et al. Long-term follow-up of IgM monoclonal gammopathy of undetermined significance. Semin Oncol. 2003;30(2):169–71.

16. Treon SP, Hunter ZR, Aggarwal A, et al. Characterization of familial Waldenstrom's macroglobulinemia. Ann Oncol. 2006;17(3):488–94.

17. McMaster ML. Familial Waldenstrom's macroglobulinemia. Semin Oncol. 2003;30(2):146–52.

18. Royer RH, Koshiol J, Giambarresi TR, et al. Differential characteristics of Waldenstrom macroglobulinemia according to patterns of familial aggregation. Blood. 2010;115(22):4464–71.

19. Aoki H, Takishita M, Kosaka M, Saito S. Frequent somatic mutations in D and/or JH segments of Ig gene in Waldenstrom's macroglobulinemia and chronic lymphocytic leukemia (CLL) with Richter's syndrome but not in common CLL. Blood. 1995;85(7):1913–9.

20. Wagner SD, Martinelli V, Luzzatto L. Similar patterns of V kappa gene usage but different degrees of somatic mutation in hairy cell leukemia, prolymphocytic leukemia, Waldenstrom's macroglobulinemia, and myeloma. Blood. 1994;83(12):3647–53.

21. Martin-Jimenez P, Garcia-Sanz R, Balanzategui A, et al. Molecular characterization of heavy chain immunoglobulin gene rearrangements in Waldenstrom's macroglobulinemia and IgM monoclonal gammopathy of undetermined significance. Haematologica. 2007;92(5):635–42.

22. Grass S, Preuss KD, Wikowicz A, et al. Hyperphosphorylated paratarg-7: a new molecularly defined risk factor for monoclonal gammopathy of undetermined significance of the IgM type and Waldenstrom macroglobulinemia. Blood. 2011;117(10):2918–23.

23. Swerdlow SH, Campo E, Harris NL, et al. WHO classification of tumours of haematopoietic and lymphoid tissues. Vol 2. 4th ed. Geneva, Switzerland: International Agency for Research on Cancer (IARC); 2008. p. 441.

24. Kyle RA, Rajkumar SV. Criteria for diagnosis, staging, risk stratification and response assessment of multiple myeloma. Leukemia. 2009;23:3–9.

25. Morice WG, Chen D, Kurtin PJ, Hanson CA, McPhail ED. Novel immunophenotypic features of marrow lymphoplasmacytic lymphoma and correlation with Waldenstrom's macroglobulinemia. Mod Pathol. 2009;22:807–16.

26. Mansoor A, Medeiros LJ, Weber DM, et al. Cytogenetic findings in lymphoplasmacytic lymphoma/Waldenstrom macroglobulinemia. Chromosomal abnormalities are associated with the polymorphous subtype and an aggressive clinical course. Am J Clin Pathol. 2001;116 (4):543–9.

27. Schop RF, Kuehl WM, Van Wier SA, et al. Waldenstrom macroglobulinemia neoplastic cells lack immunoglobulin heavy chain locus translocations but have frequent 6q deletions. Blood. 2002;100 (8):2996–3001.

28. Schop RF, Van Wier SA, Xu R, et al. 6q deletion discriminates Waldenstrom macroglobulinemia from IgM monoclonal gammopathy of undetermined significance. Cancer Genet Cytogenet. 2006;169(2):150–3.

29. Braggio E, Dogan A, Keats JJ, et al. Genomic analysis of marginal zone and lymphoplasmacytic lymphomas identified common and disease-specific abnormalities. Mod Pathol. 2012;25(5):651–60.

30. Ferreira BI, Garcia JF, Suela J, et al. Comparative genome profiling across subtypes of lowgrade B-cell lymphoma identifies type-specific and common aberrations that target genes with a role in B-cell neoplasia. Haematologica. 2008;93(5):670–9.

31. Rinaldi A, Mian M, Chigrinova E, et al. Genome-wide DNA profiling of marginal zone lymphomas identifies subtype-specific lesions with an impact on the clinical outcome. Blood. 2011;117(5):1595–604.

32. Dohner H, Stilgenbauer S, Benner A, et al. Genomic aberrations and survival in chronic lymphocytic leukemia. N Engl J Med. 2000;343 (26):1910–6.

33. Treon SP, Xu L, Yang G, et al. MYD88 L265P somatic mutation in Waldenström's macroglobulinemia. N Engl J Med. 2012;367(9):826–33.

34. Chng WJ, Schop RF, Price-Troska T, et al. Gene expression profiling of Waldenstrom macroglobulinemia reveals a phenotype more similar to chronic lymphocytic leukemia than multiple myeloma. Blood. 2006;108 (8):2755–63.

35. Gutierrez NC, Ocio EM, de Las Rivas J, et al. Gene expression profiling of B lymphocytes and plasma cells from Waldenstrom's macroglobulinemia: comparison with expression patterns of the same cell counterparts from chronic lymphocytic leukemia, multiple myeloma and normal individuals. Leukemia. 2007;21(3):541–9.

36. Hodge DR, Hurt EM, Farrar WL. The role of IL-6 and STAT3 in inflammation and cancer. Eur J Cancer. 2005;41(16):2502–12.

37. Hodge LS, Ansell SM. Jak/Stat pathway in Waldenstrom's macroglobulinemia. Clin Lymphoma Myeloma Leuk. 2011;11(1):112–4.

38. Elsawa SF, Novak AJ, Ziesmer SC, et al. Comprehensive analysis of tumor microenvironment cytokines in Waldenstrom macroglobulinemia identifies CCL5 as a novel modulator of IL-6 activity. Blood. 2011;118(20):5540–9.

39. Garcia-Sanz R, Montoto S, Torrequebrada A, et al. Waldenstrom macroglobulinemia: presenting features and outcome in a series with 217 cases. Br J Haematol. 2001;115:575–82.

40. Dimopoulos MA, Panayiotidis P, Moulopoulos LA, Sfikakis P, Dalakas M. Waldenstrom's macroglobulinemia: clinical features, complications, and management. J Clin Oncol. 2000;18(1):214–26.

41. Stone MJPV. Pathophysiology of Waldenstrom's macroglobulinemia. Haematologica. 2010;95:359–64.

42. Morel P, Duhamel A, Gobbi P, et al. International prognostic scoring system for Waldenstrom macroglobulinemia. Blood. 2009;113:4163–70.

43. Kyle RA, Treon SP, Alexanian R, et al. Prognostic markers and criteria to initiate therapy in Waldenstrom's macroglobulinemia: consensus panel recommendations from the Second International Workshop on Waldenstrom's Macroglobulinemia. Semin Oncol. 2003;30:116–20.

44. Ansell SM, Kyle RA, Reeder CB, et al. Diagnosis and management of Waldenstrom macroglobulinemia: mayo stratification of macroglobulinemia and risk-adapted therapy (mSMART) guidelines. Mayo Clin Proc. 2010;85:824–33.

45. Treon SP, Gertz MA, Dimopoulos M, et al. Update on treatment recommendations from the Third International Workshop on Waldenstrom's macroglobulinemia. Blood. 2006;107:3442–6.

46. Tedeschi A, Benevolo G, Varettoni M, et al. Fludarabine plus cyclophosphamide and rituximab in Waldenstrom macroglobulinemia: an effective but myelosuppressive regimen to be offered to patients with advanced disease. Cancer. 2012;118:434–43.

47. Treon SP, Branagan AR, Ioakimidis L, et al. Long-term outcomes to fludarabine and rituximab in Waldenstrom macroglobulinemia. Blood. 2009;113:3673–8.

48. Leleu X, Soumerai J, Roccaro A, et al. Increased incidence of transformation and myelodysplasia/acute leukemia in patients with Waldenstrom macroglobulinemia treated with nucleoside analogs. J Clin Oncol. 2009;27:250–5.

49. Annibali O, Petrucci MT, Martini V, et al. Treatment of 72 newly diagnosed Waldenstrom macroglobulinemia cases with oral melphalan, cyclophosphamide, and prednisone: results and cost analysis. Cancer. 2005;103:582–7.

50. Petrucci MT, Avvisati G, Tribalto M, Giovangrossi P, Mandelli F. Waldenstrom's macroglobulinaemia: results of a combined oral treatment in 34 newly diagnosed patients. J Intern Med. 1989;226:443–7.

51. Leblond V, Levy V, Maloisel F, et al. Multicenter, randomized comparative trial of fludarabine and the combination of cyclophosphamide-doxorubicin-prednisone in 92 patients with Waldenstrom macroglobulinemia in first relapse or with primary refractory disease. Blood. 2001;98:2640–4.

52. Tamburini J, Levy V, Chaleteix C, Fermand JP, Delmer A, Stalniewicz L, et al. Fludarabine plus cyclophosphamide in Waldenstrom's macroglobulinemia: results in 49 patients. Leukemia. 2005;19:1831–4.

53. Buske C, Hoster E, Dreyling M, et al. The addition of rituximab to front-line therapy with CHOP (R-CHOP) results in a higher response rate and longer time to treatment failure in patients with lymphoplasmacytic lymphoma: results of a randomized trial of the German Low-Grade Lymphoma Study Group (GLSG). Leukemia. 2009;23:153–61.

54. Dimopoulos MA, Anagnostopoulos A, Kyrtsonis MC, et al. Primary treatment of Waldenstrom macroglobulinemia with dexamethasone, rituximab, and cyclophosphamide. J Clin Oncol. 2007;25:3344–9.

55. Treon SP, Hanzis C, Tripsas C, et al. Bendamustine therapy in patients with relapsed or refractory Waldenstrom's macroglobulinemia. Clin Lymphoma Myeloma Leuk. 2011;11:133–5.

56. Rummel MJ, Niederle N, Maschmeyer G, et al. Bendamustine plus rituximab versus CHOP plus rituximab as first-line treatment for patients with indolent and mantle-cell lymphomas: an open-label, multicentre, randomised, phase 3 non-inferiority trial. Lancet. 2013;381(9873):1203–10.
57. Treon SP, Ioakimidis L, Soumerai JD, et al. Primary therapy of Waldenstrom macroglobulinemia with bortezomib, dexamethasone, and rituximab: WMCTG clinical trial 05-180. J Clin Oncol. 2009;27:3830–5.
58. Ghobrial IM, Xie W, Padmanabhan S, et al. Phase II trial of weekly bortezomib in combination with rituximab in untreated patients with Waldenstrom Macroglobulinemia. Am J Hematol. 2010;85:670–4.
59. Gertz MA, Rue M, Blood E, Kaminer LS, Vesole DH, Greipp PR. Multicenter phase 2 trial of rituximab for Waldenstrom macroglobulinemia (WM): an Eastern Cooperative Oncology Group Study (E3A98). Leuk Lymphoma. 2004;45:2047–55.
60. Ghobrial IM, Fonseca R, Greipp PR, et al. Initial immunoglobulin M 'flare' after rituximab therapy in patients diagnosed with Waldenstrom macroglobulinemia. Cancer. 2004;101:2593–8.
61. Kastritis E, Kyrtsonis M-C, Hatjiharissi E, et al. No significant improvement in the outcome of patients with Waldenström's macroglobulinemia treated over the last 25 years. Am J Hematol. 2011;86:479–83.
62. Davies FE, Raje N, Hideshima T, et al. Thalidomide and immunomodulatory derivatives augment natural killer cell cytotoxicity in multiple myeloma. Blood. 2001;98:210–6.
63. Treon SP, Soumerai JD, Branagan AR, et al. Thalidomide and rituximab in Waldenstrom macroglobulinemia. Blood. 2008;112:4452–7.
64. Treon SP, Soumerai JD, Branagan AR, et al. Lenalidomide and rituximab in Waldenstrom's macroglobulinemia. Clin Cancer Res. 2009;15:355–60.
65. Leleu X, Jia X, Runnels J, et al. The Akt pathway regulates survival and homing in Waldenstrom macroglobulinemia. Blood. 2007;110:4417–26.
66. Ghobrial IM, Gertz M, Laplant B, et al. Phase II trial of the oral mammalian target of rapamycin inhibitor everolimus in relapsed or refractory Waldenstrom macroglobulinemia. J Clin Oncol. 2010;28:1408–14.
67. Ghobrial IM, Poon T, Rourke M, et al. Phase II trial of single agent pabinostat (LBH589) in relapsed or relapsed/refractory Waldenstrom macroglobulinemia. San Diego: American Society of Hematology; 2010.
68. Cheson BD. Ofatumumab, a novel anti-CD20 monoclonal antibody for the treatment of B-cell malignancies. J Clin Oncol. 2010;28:3525–30.
69. Furman RR, Eradat H, DiRienzo CG, et al. A phase II trial of ofatumumab in subjects with Waldenstroms macroblobulinemia. San Diego: American Society for Hematology; 2011.
70. Treon SP, Tripsas CK, Meid K, et al. Ibrutinib in previously treated Waldenström's macroglobulinemia. N Engl J Med. 2015;372(15):1430–40.
71. Kyriakou C, Canals C, Sibon D, et al. High-dose therapy and autologous stem-cell transplantation in Waldenstrom macroglobulinemia: the lymphoma working party of the European group for blood and marrow transplantation. J Clin Oncol. 2010;28:2227–32.

72. Kyriakou C, Canals C, Cornelissen JJ, et al. Allogeneic stem-cell transplantation in patients with Waldenstrom macroglobulinemia: report from the lymphoma working party of the European group for blood and marrow transplantation. J Clin Oncol. 2010;28:4926–34.

Chapter 5
Light Chain Amyloidosis

Amara S. Hussain, MD and Anita D'Souza, MD, MS

Introduction

Light-chain (AL) amyloidosis, also known as primary systemic amyloidosis, is a rare plasma cell neoplasm. It shares with multiple myeloma the feature of clonal plasma cells but is clinically distinct from myeloma both by low tumor burden and an inherent tendency of the malignant clone to produce paraneoplastic organ damage from AL deposition. Clonal plasma cells secrete light chains that have a predisposition to misfold. The resultant misfolded and these insoluble fibrils deposit in organs leading to organ dysfunction. Light-chain amyloidosis gathers its morbidity and mortality through this spectrum of end-organ damage in vital organs such as the heart, kidneys, liver and nerves.

A.S. Hussain, MD · A. D'Souza, MD, MS (✉)
Department of Medicine, Medical College of Wisconsin,
9200W Wisconsin Avenue, Milwaukee, WI 53226, USA
e-mail: andsouza@mcw.edu

A.S. Hussain, MD
e-mail: ahussain@mcw.edu

© Springer Science+Business Media New York 2017   95
T.M. Zimmerman and S.K. Kumar (eds.),
Biology and Management of Unusual Plasma Cell Dyscrasias,
DOI 10.1007/978-1-4419-6848-7_5

Epidemiology

Light-chain amyloidosis is the most common form of systemic amyloidosis in the developed world. In Western countries, the reported incidence is approximately 1 case per 100,000 with an estimated 3000 new patients diagnosed each year in the USA. The disease shows a male predisposition (male:female ratio 2:1). The median age at diagnosis is 64 years. Patients with AL amyloidosis may have known preceding monoclonal gammopathy of undetermined significance (MGUS); AL amyloidosis accounts for 10 % of MGUS progressions. Multiple myeloma and AL amyloidosis may coexist; 10–15 % of myeloma patients have AL deposits and approximately 10 % of AL amyloidosis patients have multiple myeloma.

Pathogenesis

Pathologically, AL amyloidosis is one of several protein misfolding diseases. At the microscopic level, AL amyloid is characterized by the extracellular deposition of immunoglobulin light chains converted to anti-parallel beta-sheets that cause insoluble fibrils. Plasma cells secrete immunoglobulins which consist of heavy and light chains. In AL disease, clonal plasma cells produce an overabundance of pathogenic light chains resulting in excess free light chains in circulation. The mechanisms of conversion of these free light chains into amyloid fibrils are not fully understood but have been extensively studied in in vitro models. Factors that affect amyloid fibril formation in vitro include physicochemical factors such as temperature, pH, ionic strength, agitation, protein concentration, pressure and interactions with other ions [1].

Diagnostic Investigations

Hematologic: serum and urine protein electrophoresis with immunofixation, free light-chain assay, bone marrow biopsy.

Histologic diagnosis of amyloid deposits: Congo red stain of bone marrow and abdominal fat pad aspirate/biopsy. If both are negative, and clinical suspicion is high, proceed with biopsy of suspected organ. Sub-typing of amyloid deposits using proteomic analysis.

Detect and measure organ involvement (based on clinical suspicion)

– cardiac: troponin T, NT-proBNP, 2-dimensional echocardiogram, cardiac magnetic resonance imaging if echocardiogram is inconclusive,
– renal: 24-h urine protein, creatinine, albumin,
– hepatic: hepatomegaly (physical examination or imaging), bilirubin, alkaline phosphatase,
– neurologic: tilt table testing, electromyography and nerve conduction studies,
– gastrointestinal: fecal fat in cases of malabsorption syndrome,
– bleeding: factor X level.

Prognostication of AL Amyloidosis

A disease process with such clinical variability is difficult yet vital to prognosticate. Repeatedly, it has been shown that those patients who achieve the one-year milestone, from the date of diagnosis, have a better overall survival. To further understand this heterogeneous disease and its impact on overall survival, multiple outcome measures have been analyzed.

Early on, the degree of organ involvement, especially cardiac, underscores prognosis. Later on, the ongoing extent of light-chain clonal burden prognosticates overall survival. Table 5.1 shows factors associated with prognosis in AL amyloidosis. Cardiac involvement is the critical factor associated with early mortality. Using a NT-proBNP >1800 pg/ml, troponin T > 0.01 ng/ml and uric acid >8 mg/dl allows a prognostication of early events. The presence of none, 1, 2 or all 3 risk factors has been shown to be associated with 12, 24, 46 and 69 % risk of dying within 1 year, respectively [2]. Other prognosticators are reflective of tumor load, amyloid burden and clinical consequence of organ amyloid involvement (Table 5.1). This highlights the need for uniform and consistent use of a standard staging system for the disease as well as individual amyloid organ involvement and response to therapy, a process that was most recently revised in 2012 [3] (Table 5.2). Similarly, it is critical to define response and progression both hematologically, and in the target involved organ. Hematologic response focused on the extent of light-chain reduction. In a 2012 revision of hematologic response criteria proposed by Palladini et al. [4], complete response is defined as a negative serum and urine immunofixation electrophoresis and normal serum free light-chain ratio, very good partial response as the dFLC of less than 40 mg/L, partial response as a dFLC decrease of more than 50 % and no response. Similarly, organ response and progression are defined for key target organs such as the heart, kidneys and liver and depicted in Fig. 5.1.

Treatment

The current state of art amyloid therapies in AL amyloidosis is focused on anti-plasma cell-directed treatments. This is achieved in the form of chemotherapy that targets the underlying light-chain-secreting clone. Chemotherapy however has minimal or no effect on preformed amyloid fibrils or aggregates. These usually clear over time. As a result, there is often a lag between hematologic responses seen from reduction of the amyloidogenic clone and organ responses which needs a clearance of amyloid deposits. Often, during this time, patients, particularly those with advanced amyloidosis, can continue to worsen. Indeed, the risk of early mortality which is about 40 % in the first year after diagnosis has remained unchanged over 4 decades despite improvements in efficacy of anti-plasma cell chemotherapy [2]. Good prognostication in order to better identify the patients who are at increased risk of death or poor outcomes thus is critical.

Given that the underlying plasma cell neoplasm is similar to what is seen in multiple myeloma (albeit at a lower tumor burden), it is not surprising that AL-directed therapeutics are imported from the multiple myeloma platform. As eluded to earlier, ideal amyloid treatment would include 2 components used in conjunction:

Table 5.1 Factors associated with prognosis in AL amyloidosis

Early mortality
Cardiac troponin T [cTnT] > 0.01 ng/mL
N-terminal prohormone of brain natriuretic peptide [NT-proBNP] > 4200 pg/mL
Serum uric acid > 8 mg/dl
Plasma cell clone
Absolute measure of amyloidogenic light-chain burden (dFLC > 18 mg/dl)
Size of bone marrow plasma cells, >10 %
B_2-microglobulin
Proliferation rate of plasma cells
Presence of plasma cells in the peripheral circulation
Organs involved with amyloidosis
Number of organs involved with amyloidosis
Extent of organ involvement (e.g., the presence of symptomatic heart failure, orthostatic hypotension, etc.)
Weight loss

(a) anti-plasma cell chemotherapy (control underlying amyloido-genic clone) and (b) amyloid fibril-directed therapy (allow fibril breakdown and/or clearance). At the current time, there are no approved amyloid fibril-directed therapies, and so treatment strategies are focused on chemotherapy and intense supportive care. Figure 5.2 provides a timeline of amyloid therapeutics, and Table 5.3 further describes the various treatments that are currently tested or in testing.

Autologous Hematopoietic Cell Transplantation (Auto-transplant)

Auto-transplant using high dose melphalan chemotherapy followed by stem cell rescue is another form of plasma cell clone control. While transplant series from specialized amyloid centers have shown a benefit of auto-transplant in effective hematologic disease control and long-term survival, there is an increased risk of

Table 5.2 Staging using current definitions established in 2012 [3, 5]

Staging [6]		
Thresholds	Categories	Survival (months)
NT-proBNP > 1800 pg/ml	I (0 factors)	94.1
Troponin T > 0.025	II (1 factor)	40.3
dFLC > 18 mg/ml	III (2 factors)	14
	IV (3 factors)	5.8
Cardiac involvement		
Echo mean wall thickness > 12 mm		
NT-proBNP > 650 pg/ml		
NYHA class 3 or 4		
Histologic diagnosis		
Renal involvement		
24-h urine protein > 0.5 g/day, predominantly albumin		
Histologic diagnosis		
Hepatic involvement		
Total liver span > 15 cm (in absence of heart failure)		
Alkaline phosphatase > 1.5 times upper limit of normal		
Histologic diagnosis		
Neurologic involvement		
Peripheral nerve	Autonomic nerve	
Symmetric distal sensorimotor peripheral neuropathy	Orthostatic hypotension	
	Gastroparesis	
Histologic diagnosis	Pseudo-obstruction	
Gastrointestinal		
Macroglossia		
Histologic diagnosis in upper, mid or lower gut		
Other organs		
Cutaneous		
Carpal tunnel syndrome		
Myopathy		
Lymph node		
Arthropathy		

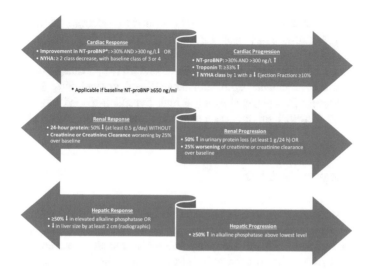

Cardiac Response
- Improvement in NT-proBNP*: >30% AND >300 ng/L↓   OR
- NYHA: ≥ 2 class decrease, with baseline class of 3 or 4

Cardiac Progression
- NT-proBNP: >30% AND >300 ng/L ↑
- Troponin T: ≥33% ↑
- ↑ NYHA class by 1 with a ↓ Ejection Fraction: ≥10%

* Applicable if baseline NT-proBNP ≥650 ng/ml

Renal Response
- 24-hour protein: 50% ↓ (at least 0.5 g/day) WITHOUT
- Creatinine or Creatinine Clearance worsening by 25% over baseline

Renal Progression
- 50% ↑ in urinary protein loss (at least 1 g/24 h) OR
- 25% worsening of creatinine or creatinine clearance over baseline

Hepatic Response
- ≥50% ↓ in elevated alkaline phosphatase OR
- ↓ in liver size by at least 2 cm (radiographic)

Hepatic Progression
- ≥50% ↑ in alkaline phosphatase above lowest level

Fig. 5.1 Definitions of organ response and progression

transplant-related mortality particularly among patients with advanced disease. In 2007, the results of a much anticipated randomized control clinical trial comparing auto-transplant to oral chemotherapy (melphalan/dexamethasone) failed to show a survival benefit with auto-transplant compared to oral chemotherapy [8]. However, several issues were raised regarding this study including several patients in the auto-transplant arm not getting planned transplants, lowering of melphalan conditioning dose in a third of transplanted patients, and an exceedingly high mortality of 24 % in the transplant arm which in part was likely related to patients with advanced cardiac involvement and may be a center experience. Prognostic factors related to increased early mortality post-transplant and poor overall survival include a poor pre-transplant performance score (Karnofsky <80 %), advanced cardiac involvement (NYHA 3 or 4, EF <40 %), biomarkers, NT-proBNP > 5000, troponin T > 0.06, more than 3 organ involvement with AL and severe autonomic neuropathy. The use of these criteria to guide transplant eligibility has lowered the risk of early mortality. Indeed, improved patient selection and supportive care have led to decreasing rates of post-transplant mortality and translated into improved overall survival in a large transplant series of over 1500 patients reported to the Center for International Blood and Marrow Transplant Research (CIBMTR) [9]. Allogeneic transplant has been reported in individual case reports and small series. The European Group of Blood and Marrow Transplantation reported 19 patients with allogeneic transplant (including 4 with syngeneic transplant) showing a high transplant-related mortality of 40 % with 7 survivors at a median follow-up of 19 months [10].

Supportive Care

Good supportive care is essential in the care of amyloid patients. AL patients have unique clinical problems. For e.g., patients are at an increased risk of becoming volume overload; however, over diuresis leading to even mild intravascular depletion can precipitate gastrointestinal upset, including nausea and vomiting, or worse, induce cardiorenal syndrome. As a result, diuresis and albumin infusions may be necessary to achieve euvolemia. Patients with orthostatic hypotension may need midodrine and fludrocortisone. However, fludrocortisone can worsen fluid retention. Other complications that may be more amplified in AL patients include bleeding (gastrointestinal), cardiac arrhythmias and unresponsive hypotension. Table 5.4 provides examples of supportive care that is often needed. This again highlights the need for a multi-disciplinary team approach while caring for these patients.

Solid Organ Transplant in AL Amyloidosis

The UNOS data in both renal and cardiac transplant suggest poor outcomes in amyloidosis (regardless of amyloid sub-type) [11, 12]; however, there may be a role for organ transplant in AL amyloidosis. A concern for recurrence of the amyloid process in the transplanted organ, in the setting of an incurable underlying clonal disease, is not to be understated. Sequential transplant in select patients with limited organ burden outside of the organ to be transplanted may be attempted either following chemotherapy or

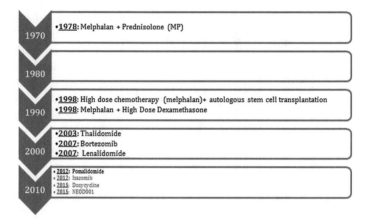

Fig. 5.2 Timeline of therapies (when the therapy was first described in the literature. Therapies marked in *red* imply drugs in active testing)

with an adjuvant autologous hematopoietic cell transplantation post-organ transplant. This has been reported with varying success from high-volume specialized amyloid centers such as the National Amyloid Center in the United Kingdom, Mayo Clinic and Boston University in cardiac and renal organ transplants.

The Future of AL Therapies

Results of clinical trials testing newer agents in a randomized controlled setting including bortezomib (melphalan/dexamethasone versus bortezomib/melphalan/dexamethasone, NCT01277016) and ixazomib (ixazomib compared to investigator choice in relapsed AL amyloidosis, NCT01659658) are eagerly anticipated. The role of auto-transplant needs to be re-defined in the current era of improved selection criteria and novel therapies. With refinements in transplant eligibility and lowering of transplant-related mortality, it may be time to re-consider a randomized clinical trial comparing transplant versus non-transplant approaches with novel chemotherapies. Finally, there is excitement over anti-fibril-directed therapies with agents such as NEOD001 entering the clinical phase testing (NCT02312206).

Table 5.3 Selected key therapies in AL amyloidosis

Regimen	Mechanism	Strength of data	Adverse events	Other consideration
Melphalan/Dexamethasone	Alkylator	Phase II, III	Cytopenias	Generally well tolerated (elderly, advanced cardiac involvement)
			Risk of myelodysplasia	Not stem cell sparing
			Nausea	Slow response
				Only regimen shown to have efficacy in randomized clinical trial
Thalidomide	Immunomodulatory	Phase II	Fluid retention and cardiac issues: progression of congestive heart failure, increase of biomarkers, and arrhythmias	Stem cell sparing
				Combination cyclophosphamide–thalidomide–dexamethasone
Bortezomib	Proteasome inhibitor	Phase I/II	Neuropathy	Administer via SQ to ↓ toxicity
			Concern for worsening cardiac function in patients with advanced cardiac involvement [7].	Common combination: cyclophosphamide/bortezomib/dexamethasone based on retrospective data
			GI toxicity	

(continued)

Table 5.3 (continued)

Regimen	Mechanism	Strength of data	Adverse events	Other consideration
Lenalidomide	Immunomodulatory drug	Phase II	Cytopenias	Not stem cell sparing
			GI toxicity	Relapsed setting
			Fatigue	Dose reduction in renal failure
			Skin toxicity	
Pomalidomide	Immunemodulatory	Phase II	Cytopenias	Relapsed setting
			Fatigue	
Ixazomib	Proteasome inhibitor	Phase III ongoing	GI toxicity	Oral regimen
			Skin toxicity	
Doxycycline	Amyloid fibril breakdown (?)	Phase II ongoing	Generally safe	In conjunction with chemotherapy Localized amyloidosis (?)
NEOD001	Amyloid fibril clearance	Phase I	?	In conjunction with chemotherapy
		Phase III underway		

Table 5.4 Supportive care in treatment of AL amyloidosis

	Helpful
Fluid retention and weight gain	Loop diuretics, spironolactone
	Periodic pleurocentesis may be needed
	May be worsened by salt tablets, fludrocortisone often used in orthostatic hypotension
Heart failure	Diuretics
	Salt and fluid restriction
	Caution with calcium channel blockers, digoxin (can bind to amyloid fibrils leading to digoxin toxicity), beta blockers may cause decompensation
	Afterload reduction (ACE-I, ARBs) poorly tolerated
Cardiac arrhythmias (atrial fibrillation, ventricular arrhythmias, Sudden Cardiac Death)	Amiodarone
	AV nodal ablation and pacemaker
	AICD in select patients may be considered
	Caution with rate lowering agents such as calcium channel blockers, beta blockers, digoxin
Orthostatic hypotension	Waist-high elastic stockings
	Midodrine
	Salt tablets, fludrocortisone (can worsen fluid retention)
	Continuous noradrenalin infusion (for refractory hypotension)
Neuropathic pain	Gabapentin
	Pregabalin
	Duloxetine
	Amitriptyline
	Nortriptyline
	Topical agents (lidocaine, TCA, ketamine)
Nephrotic syndrome	Diuretics
	Low-dose ACE-I (if patient is not hypotensive)

Table 5.4 (continued)

	Helpful
Renal failure	Dialysis
	Patients may need pre-transplant midodrine (particularly in those with autonomic neuropathy)
Gastroparesis causing nausea and vomiting	Anti-emetics, metoclopramide
Intestinal pseudo-obstruction	Neostigmine
Diarrhea	Fiber supplements
	Bile salt binding agents
	Loperamide
	Octreotide (in refractory cases)
Malnutrition	Dietician consultation early
	Parenteral nutrition may be needed in those with severe steatorrhea
Anti-coagulation	May be needed in patients with cardiomyopathy, atrial fibrillation
	Check factor X levels
	Higher risk of GI bleeding

References

1. Baden EM, Sikkink LA, Ramirez-Alvarado M. Light chain amyloidosis—Current findings and future prospects. Curr Protein Pept Sci. 2009;10:500–8.
2. Kumar SK, Gertz MA, Lacy MQ, et al. Recent improvements in survival in primary systemic amyloidosis and the importance of an early mortality risk score. Mayo Clin Proc. 2011;86:12–8.
3. Comenzo RL, Reece D, Palladini G, et al. Consensus guidelines for the conduct and reporting of clinical trials in systemic light-chain amyloidosis. Leukemia. 2012;26:2317–25.
4. Palladini G, Dispenzieri A, Gertz MA, et al. New criteria for response to treatment in immunoglobulin light chain amyloidosis based on free light chain measurement and cardiac biomarkers: impact on survival outcomes. J Clin Oncol. 2012;30:4541–9.
5. Dispenzieri A, Gertz MA, Buadi F. What do I need to know about immunoglobulin light chain (AL) amyloidosis? Blood Rev. 2012;26:137–54.
6. Kumar S, Dispenzieri A, Lacy MQ, et al. Revised prognostic staging system for light chain amyloidosis incorporating cardiac biomarkers and serum free light chain measurements. J Clin Oncol. 2012;30:989–95.

7. Hussain A, et al. Am J Hematol. 2015;90(11):E212–3.
 8. Jaccard A, Moreau P, Leblond V, et al. High-dose melphalan versus melphalan plus dexamethasone for AL amyloidosis. N Engl J Med. 2007;357:1083–93.
 9. D'Souza A, Dispenzieri A, Wirk B, et al. Improved outcomes after autologous hematopoietic cell transplantation for light chain amyloidosis: a Center for International Blood and Marrow Transplantation Research study. J Clin Oncol. 2015;33(32):3741–9.
10. Schonland SO, Lokhorst H, Buzyn A, et al. Allogeneic and syngeneic hematopoietic cell transplantation in patients with amyloid light-chain amyloidosis: a report from the European Group for Blood and Marrow Transplantation. Blood. 2006;107:2578–84.
11. Bradshaw SH, Veinot JP. Cardiac amyloidosis: what are the indications for transplant? Curr Opin Cardiol. 2012;27:143–7.
12. Bleyer AJ, Donaldson LA, McIntosh M, et al. Relationship between underlying renal disease and renal transplantation outcome. Am J Kidney Dis. 2001;37:1152–61.

Chapter 6
Immunoglobulin Deposition Diseases

Vinay Gupta, MD, Wilson I. Gonsalves, MD and Francis K. Buadi, MB, ChB

Introduction

Monoclonal immunoglobulins may be associated with a variety of renal diseases as a result of direct deposition of the monoclonal immunoglobulin and also from an indirect mechanism via dysregulation of the alternative pathway of complement. A thorough and complete clinical evaluation of the patient is required prior to categorizing their renal disease as related to the monoclonal protein. Tissue biopsy is essential for the diagnosis, and the initial workup should also include quantification and identification of monoclonal proteins with serum protein electrophoresis (SPEP), urine protein electrophoresis (UPEP), immunofixation (IFE), and quantitative serum light-chain assay. However, some may also present without evidence of a circulating paraprotein. Furthermore,

V. Gupta, MD · W.I. Gonsalves, MD · F.K. Buadi, MB, ChB (✉)
Division of Hematology, Department of Medicine, Mayo Clinic, 200 First
St. SW, Rochester, MN 55905, USA
e-mail: buadi.francis@mayo.edu

W.I. Gonsalves, MD
e-mail: gonsalves.wilson@mayo.edu

© Springer Science+Business Media New York 2017
T.M. Zimmerman and S.K. Kumar (eds.),
Biology and Management of Unusual Plasma Cell Dyscrasias,
DOI 10.1007/978-1-4419-6848-7_6

in a significant proportion of patients, with a detected circulating monoclonal paraprotein, the end-organ pathology may not be directly attributable to monoclonal gammopathy making a directed biopsy of the kidney essential in establishing the diagnosis [33].

This chapter will review the clinical presentation and management of a spectrum of rare monoclonal gammopathy-associated renal lesions such as: monoclonal immunoglobulin deposition disease (MIDD), Type I cryoglobulinemia, proliferative glomerulonephritis with monoclonal IgG deposits (PGNMID), C3 monoclonal-associated glomerulonephritis, immunotactoid glomerulonephropathy (ITG), light-chain proximal tubulopathy (LCPT) or Fanconi's syndrome and light-chain crystallopathy. Myeloma-related cast nephropathy and renal disease secondary to systemic light-chain amyloidosis will not be discussed in this chapter.

Monoclonal Immunoglobulin Deposition Disease (MIDD)

MIDD is a systemic disorder characterized by tissue deposition of monoclonal immunoglobulin protein. An underlying plasma cell proliferative disorder is responsible for production and secretion of these immunoglobulin chain fragments, leading to their deposition into vital organs such as kidneys, heart, and liver, resulting in organ dysfunction. Depending on the component or fragment of the immunoglobulin that is deposited, MIDD is divided into light-chain deposition disease (LCDD), heavy-chain deposition disease (HCDD), or mixed light- and heavy-chain deposition disease (LHCDD). Although, MIDD remains a rare disease with an estimated annual incidence of 8 cases per million [22], large retrospective case series and database analyses have attempted to improve our understanding of the disease. In the largest case series of 64 patients with pathologically verified renal MIDD [31], a majority of patients carried a diagnosis of LCDD (80 %; 51 of 64), followed by 7 patients with HCDD and 6 patients with LHCDD.

Clinical Presentation and Course

Most of the clinical data on MIDD are based on reports of patients with LCDD. The median age of patients is around 50–60 years which is significantly lower than other plasma cell dyscrasias. The incidence is higher in men as compared to women. They tend to present in an insidious fashion; however, cases of rapid progression manifested by rapid organ dysfunction have been described. The most common site of immunoglobulin deposition is the kidneys, presenting with progressive decline in glomerular function leading to renal insufficiency, albuminuria which often reaches nephrotic range, hypertension, and hematuria. In the absence of timely initiation of therapy, renal dysfunction progresses to ESRD [17], and in a small but significant number of patients, ESRD requiring renal replacement therapy is the presenting feature. Cardiac involvement is relatively less frequent and may be symptomatic with findings consistent with congestive heart failure and life-threatening arrhythmias [38]. The plasma cell burden is low in MIDD and does not meet criteria for diagnosis of MM [11]. Additionally, cytogenetic abnormalities associated with MM are rare in MIDD [11]. Other organ systems that may be involved include the liver, lungs, and nervous system. The degree of hepatic involvement ranges from mild transaminitis to portal hypertension and liver failure [38].

In LCDD, light microscopy demonstrates monoclonal protein deposits along glomerular and tubular basement membrane resembling nodular glomerulosclerosis (Fig. 6.1). Immunofluorescence (IF) reveals clonality of deposited immunoglobulin light chains (Fig. 6.2). On electron microscopy (EM), the deposits appear granular and unorganized in nature. The light chains are predominantly κ in nature in up to 85 % cases [22]. In contrast to amyloidosis, LCDD does not show a β-pleated folding configuration or fibrillar pattern and does not stain positive with Congo red or show apple green birefringence under polarized light [22]. In HCDD, either complete heavy-chain or truncated heavy-chain immunoglobulins are deposited into tissues, often along with light-chain fragments. The heavy chains are composed of γ isotype [31]. As in LCDD, HCDD is distinguished from AH amyloidosis by non-fibrillar deposits and negative Congo red staining.

The prognosis of MIDD is dependent upon various factors, such as degree of renal and cardiac involvement, age, clinical comorbidity, and timeliness of initiation of therapy. Length of survival, therefore, ranges widely across various case series, with a median of 4 years [27]. In a case series of 63 patients, factors independently associated with poor prognosis and inferior survival in LCDD included increased age at presentation, coexisting plasma cell proliferative disorder, and extrarenal light-chain deposition [35].

Treatment

Given rarity of disease, no randomized trial data are available to establish standard of care. The primary goal of therapy is to abrogate production of immunoglobulin light chains and prevent further renal damage. Essentially, this translates into administration of therapy directed at elimination of the underlying clonal plasma cells, which are typically associated with a low proliferative index.

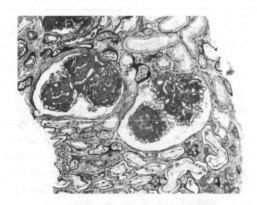

Fig. 6.1 A case of LCDD shows nodular mesangial sclerosis and thickening of tubular basement membranes. The monoclonal protein deposits in the mesangium and tubular basement membranes are positive for periodic acid–Schiff stain (X 400)

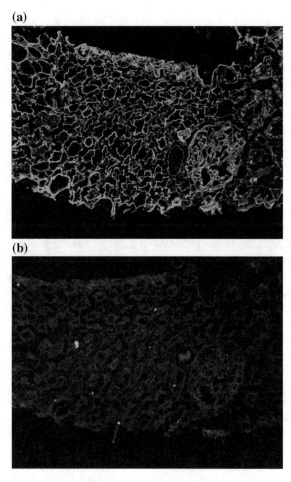

Fig. 6.2 Immunofluorescence on a case of lambda type LCDD shows diffuse linear glomerular and tubular basement membranes positivity for lambda (**a**) with negative kappa (**b**) (X200)

Currently, the use of induction-based chemotherapy followed by consolidation with an autologous stem cell transplant if appropriate is the favored approach of managing such patients.

The combination of melphalan and prednisone remained a frontline agent in the management of LCDD for years. In appropriate candidates, consolidation therapy with stem cell transplantation is associated with acceptable toxicity and improved long-term outcomes as opposed to chemotherapy alone [40, 50]. Improvements in renal function after ASCT have been reported, with reversal of dialysis dependence in one report [10, 50]. Weichman et al. [50] reported a case series of six patients with LCDD, who underwent ASCT with melphalan-based conditioning. Five of total six patients achieved a complete hematological remission (CHR), which was maintained at a median follow-up of 12 months. Encouragingly, improvement in renal function was also noted [50]. In another single-center retrospective analysis of six patients, high-dose chemotherapy followed by ASCT achieved both hematological and renal response [23]. Similarly, another report from Telio et al. [46] retrospectively reviewed eight patients with LCDD or LHCDD who underwent ASCT with melphalan-based conditioning regimen resulting in high rates of hematological and renal response.

Novel agents such as proteasome inhibitors may also be especially useful in this disease, as they are effective in patients with plasma cell dyscrasias presenting with renal insufficiency. Kastritis et al. reported the use of combination of bortezomib and dexamethasone as induction regimen in four patients with LCDD resulting in partial response in two and complete response in the other two patients. Of these, three patients proceeded to ASCT with melphalan-based conditioning and achieved a CHR at last follow-up [20]. Recently, Tovar et al. have reported the use of combination of bortezomib and dexamethasone as induction therapy followed by ASCT in three patients, of which two achieved a complete response (CR) with last follow-up at 34 and 40 months [48].

End-organ dysfunction and damage necessitates appropriate supportive care. Given near universal renal involvement, renal replacement therapy in the form of dialysis may be needed. The role of renal transplantation is unclear [22]. Median allograft survival in patients with LCDD is low secondary to recurrence of primary disease in the transplanted kidney. In a retrospective analysis, 71 % of patients were noted to have recurrence LCCD leading to a median graft survival of only 37.5 months, which is significantly lower than the decade or longer survival seen in non-LCDD patients [22]. Given poor allograft survival, selection of appropriate patients for renal transplantation is necessary.

Patients who achieve a complete hematological response with residual renal dysfunction may be appropriate candidates in this regard. Close surveillance and institution of further therapy as needed to prevent production and deposition of monoclonal immunoglobulins is needed to justify allocation of donor organs.

Type I Cryoglobulinemia

Cryoglobulinemia is characterized by the presence of cryoglobulins which are serum proteins that tend to precipitate under conditions of cold exposure. The broquet classification, based on the clonality of involved immunoglobulins, classifies cryoglobulinemia into Type I (monoclonal; commonly IgG or IgM), Type II (both monoclonal and polyclonal), and Type III (polyclonal) [4].

Type I cryoglobulinemia is associated with clonal plasma cell or B-cell disorder, commonly MM or Waldenstrom's macroglobulinemia.

Clinical Presentation and Course

The majority of patients with Type I CG remain asymptomatic. Depending on the degree of cryoglobulinemia and offending factors, patients may present with sequelae of thrombosis characteristically manifesting as Raynaud phenomenon, acral cyanosis, and ischemia or with symptoms of hyperviscosity such as blurred vision, headache, diplopia, and confusion. Cryoglobulinemia, however, has protean manifestations, and the involvement of other organ systems such as cutaneous, pulmonary, renal, and musculoskeletal structures is common. Of these, renal involvement presents as membranoproliferative glomerulonephritis with microtubular deposits composed of monoclonal cryoglobulin [19].

Treatment

The management of cryoglobulinemia relies heavily on patient education and close monitoring for complications. Limiting cold exposure is encouraged. The treatment of underlying plasma cell or lymphoproliferative disorder may be required if preventive measures are inadequate. The general paradigm of managing cryoglobulinemia is to direct treatment against the underlying cause leading to the formation of cryoglobulins. It is also important to gauge the severity of the cryoglobulinemia symptoms when choosing an appropriate therapeutic regimen. For mild symptoms such as purpura, arthralgias, or mild neuropathy, observation, avoidance of cold temperatures, or wearing warm clothing should suffice.

Type I cryoglobulinemia should be managed with therapies directed against eradicating the underlying clonal cells responsible for producing the offending immunoglobulin. In cases secondary to overt neoplastic disorders such as MM, non-Hodgkin's lymphoma, or Waldenstrom's macroglobulinemia, established chemotherapeutic regimens for each of those respective malignant conditions should be utilized to halt the production of cryoglobulins [13, 34, 41]. In one series, high-dose melphalan chemotherapy was utilized in four patients with Type I cryoglobulinemia due to MM, all of whom derived disease control for at least 18 months or more [34]. However, more indolent clonal processes such as MGUS can be treated with agents ranging from corticosteroids or alkylating agents [9, 47]. Novel biological agents such as bortezomib, thalidomide, and lenalidomide may be used in severe and/or refractory patients [2, 5, 9, 32, 47].

Patients with life-threatening vasculitis including cryoglobulinemic nephropathy, skin ulcers, or symptoms related to hyperviscosity may require the use of plasmapheresis to help reduce the levels of circulating cryoglobulin complexes [37, 43, 45]. However, this does not treat the underlying disease and is unable to achieve long-term disease control. Furthermore, there can be rebound elevation in cryoglobulin production after the cessation of plasmapheresis [7]. Thus, cytotoxic therapy must be instituted concurrently to help maintain disease control.

Proliferative Glomerulonephritis with Monoclonal IgG Deposits (PGNMID)

PGNMID is a distinct entity that resembles immune complex-mediated glomerulonephritis except that immunoglobulin deposits are comprised of intact monoclonal immunoglobulins [29].

Clinical Presentation and Course

The most common clinical features include varying degrees of hematuria, renal insufficiency, hypertension, and nephrotic syndrome. A low serum C3 level can also be present. The kidney biopsy typically shows a membranoproliferative pattern of injury in most cases. On immunofluorescence, monoclonal immunoglobulins deposits are seen in the mesangial and capillary wall. If the heavy chain consists of IgG, subtyping the IgG commonly finds the IgG3 subclass [30]. In the Nasr study, a monoclonal serum protein was detected at presentation in 30 % of patients, only one patient had multiple myeloma; however, none of rest of the patients went on to develop an overt hematological malignancy. In 32 patients for which extended follow-up was available, complete response (CR) as defined by remission of proteinuria to <500 mg/d with normal renal function was noted in 4 and partial response (PR) as defined by reduction in proteinuria by at least 50 % with stable renal function in 8 patients, while progression to ESRD was noted in 7 patients.

Treatment

There is no standard treatment for PGNMID. In one case series, 18 patients received immunomodulatory drugs, 9 received angiotensin-converting enzyme inhibitors (ACE) or angiotensin II receptor blockers (ARB), 3 received alkylating agents, 1 each received bortezomib or combination of bortezomib and thalidomide, while 5 patients were not treated. Patients demonstrating at least a PR or better were seen in 8 of 18 patients who received immunomodulatory agents and 4 of 9 patients who received an ACEi or an ARB [30]. If the offending monoclonal immunoglobulin detected on a renal biopsy is also detected in serum or urine or both, we prefer to combine bortezomib, cyclophosphamide, and dexamethasone for IgG and IgA monoclonal proteins and rituximab alone or in combination with cyclophosphamide and dexamethasone for IgM monoclonal proteins.

C3 Monoclonal-Associated Glomerulonephritis

C3 monoclonal-associated glomerulonephritis (C3 GN) is characterized by proliferative glomerulonephritis in response to aberrant glomerular deposition of complement factors secondary to functional inhibition of complement regulatory pathways by monoclonal paraproteins [51]. The hallmark pathological finding is intense C3 staining without evidence of concomitant immunoglobulin deposition.

Clinical Presentation

In a retrospective review of 32 patients by Zand et al., the clinical course was variable reflecting the heterogeneous nature of the disease. Despite aggressive workup, only 10 (31 %) had a serum monoclonal protein, of these 1 patient was identified to have chronic lymphocytic leukemia, while the rest were classified as MGUS. One patient, who underwent a kidney transplant, developed pathological evidence of recurrent C3 GN on follow-up biopsy of the graft, suggesting the importance of controlling the underlying clonal cell disorder.

Treatment

In many cases, the condition remains indolent and requires no therapy. However, in the setting of progressive renal dysfunction, steroids or steroids in combination with cyclophosphamide can be used in patients with no detectable monoclonal protein. There is no clear evidence of the benefit of immunomodulatory agents, proteasome inhibitors, or alkylator-based regimens in the management of C3 GN. However, in patients who have an IgG or IgA monoclonal protein with rapidly progressive disease not responsive to steroids alone or steroid in combination with cyclophosphamide, bortezomib in combination with cytoxan and dexamethasone has been used. Furthermore, for IgM monoclonal protein, rituximab alone or in combination with cyclophosphamide and dexamethasone can be used. Within this context, interventions are dictated by the clinical picture and close follow-up remains important. Targeting the complement system remains an active area of research.

Immunotactoid Glomerulonephropathy (ITG)

ITG is an extremely rare disorder associated with a monoclonal gammopathy, as exemplified by an incidence rate of ~ 0.06 % based on 10,108 native kidney biopsies [39]. It is characterized by proliferative glomerulonephritis on light microscopy, IgG deposits on immunofluorescence microscopy, and focal intraglomerular deposition of non-amyloid microfibrils or microtubules, usually >30 nm in diameter and arranged in parallel or stacked arrays as seen on electron microscopy. It is important to distinguish ITG from the more common fibrillary glomerulonephritis (FGN), which is associated with polyclonal immunoglobulin deposits and lack of association with underlying plasma cell and lymphoproliferative disorder.

Clinical Presentation

Clinically, hematuria, renal insufficiency, hypertension, and nephrotic syndrome are commonly seen in patients with ITG [36]. Extrarenal involvement is rarely seen in these patients. The common hematological malignancies associated with ITG are chronic

lymphocytic   leukemia,   myeloma,   and   lymphoplasmacytic
lymphoma.

Treatment

The management strategy is aimed at treating the underlying
hematological process. Given rarity of disease, no clear outcome
with specific agents is identified. Reports have demonstrated that
one patient with underlying chronic lymphocytic leukemia did
have a response to treatment with fludarabine-based regimen with
decreased proteinuria and improvement in renal function.
Cadaveric renal transplantation has been performed in these
patients with maintenance of the allograft function for significant
duration despite ITG recurrence in the transplanted kidney.

Light-Chain Proximal Tubulopathy (LCPT) or Fanconi Syndrome

LCPT is the most common subtype of crystal-storing histiocytosis
disorders which are a group of monoclonal gammopathy disorders
characterized by lysosomal processing and intracellular deposition
of crystallized immunoglobulin free light chains in the kidneys,
and other organ systems, such as the spleen, liver, and bone marrow, may also be involved [25].

Clinical Presentation

In LCPT, the disease is localized to the proximal renal tubular
epithelium and extrarenal manifestations are rare [42]. The
underlying plasma cell dyscrasia is commonly low-grade MM or
MGUS [24] secreting immunoglobulin light chains [26]. It is rarely
associated with LPL [3, 49]. The clinical presentation is consistent
with defects in sodium-coupled cellular co-transport mechanisms.

This is then seen clinically as Type II renal tubular acidosis, aminoaciduria, glycosuria, and phosphaturia [42]. Urinary loss of phosphorus leads to increase in parathyroid hormone and resultant vitamin D-resistant osteomalacia, often presenting as microscopic bone fractures and bone pain [11, 16, 26].

Treatment

The optimal therapy is unknown; however, institution of therapy directed at the underlying hematological disorder may be required in a small number of patients. Recently, stem cell transplantation has been utilized with good success in stabilization or improvement of the renal function in LCPT patients. Fortunately, the rate of progression to ESRD or symptomatic multiple myeloma remains low. Furthermore, measures to ameliorate further bone loss include calcium, phosphate, and vitamin D supplementation [6].

Light-Chain Crystallopathy

The crystallization and subsequent deposition of monoclonal paraproteins into systemic vasculature is exceedingly rare, with less than fifty reported cases in literature [1, 8, 14, 15, 18, 21, 28, 44]. Among these, an underlying plasma cell dyscrasia, most commonly MM, is often identified. However, there are no clearly identified risk factors in myeloma patients who are predisposed to crystallopathy.

Clinical Symptoms

Crystalglobulin deposition injures and activates the vascular endothelium, thus triggering procoagulant mechanisms, ultimately leading to thrombosis and consequent vascular compromise leading to end-organ damage. The renal vasculature is most commonly involved and often presents as sudden decline in renal function, which is often irreversible. Less appreciated are the cutaneous, ocular, neurological, and musculoskeletal complications. Biopsy of the involved organ, commonly kidneys and skin, is required to establish the diagnosis.

Treatment

Despite rarity of the condition, crystal-induced glomerulopathy should be included in the differential diagnosis, as directed and timely therapy to reduce monoclonal paraproteinemia in the form of plasmapheresis and high-dose steroids may prevent or reverse renal dysfunction and also serve as bridging therapy for definitive therapy. The mainstay of therapy remains treatment of the underlying plasma cell disorder. There is no clear evidence for efficacy of alkylator-based therapy. Hashimoto et al. reported resolution of cutaneous ulcers and partial correction of renal dysfunction in a patient treated with thalidomide- and dexamethasone-based therapy [15]. We have recently employed a bortezomib-based approach with encouraging results in one patient, with stabilization of renal dysfunction and complete resolution of cutaneous ulceration [12].

Conclusion

Renal diseases associated with monoclonal gammopathy are the result of a toxic monoclonal protein produced by lymphoid-derived hematopoietic cells such as B cells or plasma cells. These disorders rarely require treatment to prevent their progression to overt malignancy, but urgent therapy is sometime required to prevent deterioration of renal complications. A thorough and complete clinical evaluation that may involve a renal biopsy must be performed in every patient suspected of having their renal disease related to a monoclonal gammopathy.

Acknowledgments We thank Dr. Samih H. Nasr for providing the images used in this manuscript.

References

1. Ball NJ, Wickert W, et al. Crystalglobulinemia syndrome. A manifestation of multiple myeloma. Cancer. 1993;71(4):1231–4.
2. Besada E, Vik A, et al. Successful treatment with bortezomib in type-1 cryoglobulinemic vasculitis patient after rituximab failure: a case report and literature review. Int J Hematol. 2013;97(6):800–3.
3. Bridoux F, Sirac C, et al. Fanconi's syndrome induced by a monoclonal Vkappa3 light chain in Waldenstrom's macroglobulinemia. Am J Kidney Dis. 2005;45(4):749–57.
4. Brouet JC, Clauvel JP, et al. Biologic and clinical significance of cryoglobulins. A report of 86 cases. Am J Med. 1974;57(5):775–88.
5. Cem Ar M, Soysal T, et al. Successful management of cryoglobulinemia-induced leukocytoclastic vasculitis with thalidomide in a patient with multiple myeloma. Ann Hematol. 2005;84(9):609–13.
6. Clarke BL, Wynne AG, et al. Osteomalacia associated with adult Fanconi's syndrome: clinical and diagnostic features. Clin Endocrinol (Oxf). 1995;43 (4):479–90.
7. Dispenzieri A. Symptomatic cryoglobulinemia. Curr Treat Options Oncol. 2000;1(2):105–18.
8. Dotten DA, Pruzanski W, et al. Cryocrystalglobulinemia. Can Med Assoc J. 1976;114(10):909–12.
9. Fermand JP, Bridoux F, et al. How I treat monoclonal gammopathy of renal significance (MGRS). Blood. 2013;122(22):3583–90.
10. Firkin F, Hill PA, et al. Reversal of dialysis-dependent renal failure in light-chain deposition disease by autologous peripheral blood stem cell transplantation. Am J Kidney Dis. 2004;44(3):551–5.
11. Gertz MA. Managing light chain deposition disease. Leuk Lymphoma. 2012;53(2):183–4.
12. Gupta V, El Ters M, et al. Crystalglobulin-induced nephropathy. J Am Soc Nephrol JASN. 2015;26(3):525–9.
13. Harel S, Mohr M, et al. Clinico-biological characteristics and treatment of type I monoclonal cryoglobulinaemia: a study of 64 cases. Br J Haematol. 2015;168(5):671–8.
14. Hasegawa H, Ozawa T, et al. Multiple myeloma-associated systemic vasculopathy due to crystalglobulin or polyarteritis nodosa. Arthritis Rheum. 1996;39(2):330–4.
15. Hashimoto R, Toda T, et al. Abnormal N-glycosylation of the immunoglobulin G kappa chain in a multiple myeloma patient with crystalglobulinemia: case report. Int J Hematol. 2007;85(3):203–6.
16. Hashimoto T, Arakawa K, et al. Acquired Fanconi syndrome with osteomalacia secondary to monoclonal gammopathy of undetermined significance. Intern Med. 2007;46(5):241–5.
17. Heilman RL, Velosa JA, et al. Long-term follow-up and response to chemotherapy in patients with light-chain deposition disease. Am J Kidney Dis. 1992;20(1):34–41.

18. Kanno Y, Okada H, et al. Crystal nephropathy: a variant form of myeloma kidney—A case report and review of the literature. Clin Nephrol. 2001;56 (5):398–401.

19. Karras A, Noel LH, et al. Renal involvement in monoclonal (type I) cryoglobulinemia: two cases associated with IgG3 kappa cryoglobulin. Am J Kidney Dis. 2002;40(5):1091–6.

20. Kastritis E, Migkou M, et al. Treatment of light chain deposition disease with bortezomib and dexamethasone. Haematologica. 2009;94(2):300–2.

21. Langlands DR, Dawkins RL, et al. Arthritis associated with a crystallizing cryoprecipitable IgG paraprotein. Am J Med. 1980;68(3):461–5.

22. Leung N, Lager DJ, et al. Long-term outcome of renal transplantation in light-chain deposition disease. Am J Kidney Dis. 2004;43(1):147–53.

23. Lorenz EC, Gertz MA, et al. Long-term outcome of autologous stem cell transplantation in light chain deposition disease. Nephrol Dial Transplant. 2008;23(6):2052–7.

24. Maldonado JE, Velosa JA, et al. Fanconi syndrome in adults. A manifestation of a latent form of myeloma. Am J Med. 1975;58 (3):354–64.

25. Merlini G, Stone MJ. Dangerous small B-cell clones. Blood. 2006;108 (8):2520–30.

26. Messiaen T, Deret S, et al. Adult Fanconi syndrome secondary to light chain gammopathy. Clinicopathologic heterogeneity and unusual features in 11 patients. Medicine (Baltimore). 2000;79(3):135–54.

27. Montseny JJ, Kleinknecht D, et al. Long-term outcome according to renal histological lesions in 118 patients with monoclonal gammopathies. Nephrol Dial Transplant. 1998;13(6):1438–45.

28. Mullen B, Chalvardjian A. Crystalline tissue deposits on a case of multiple myeloma. Arch Pathol Lab Med. 1981;105(2):94–7.

29. Nasr SH, Markowitz GS, et al. Proliferative glomerulonephritis with monoclonal IgG deposits: a distinct entity mimicking immune-complex glomerulonephritis. Kidney Int. 2004;65(1):85–96.

30. Nasr SH, Satoskar A, et al. Proliferative glomerulonephritis with monoclonal IgG deposits. J Am Soc Nephrol JASN. 2009;20(9):2055–64.

31. Nasr SH, Valeri AM, et al. Renal monoclonal immunoglobulin deposition disease: a report of 64 patients from a single institution. Clin J Am Soc Nephrol. 2012;7(2):231–9.

32. Ninomiya S, Fukuno K, et al. IgG type multiple myeloma and concurrent IgA type monoclonal gammopathy of undetermined significance complicated by necrotizing skin ulcers due to type I cryoglobulinemia. J Clin Exp Hematopathol JCEH. 2010;50(1):71–4.

33. Paueksakon P, Revelo MP, et al. Monoclonal gammopathy: significance and possible causality in renal disease. Am J Kidney Dis. 2003;42(1):87–95.

34. Payet J, Livartowski J, et al. Type I cryoglobulinemia in multiple myeloma, a rare entity: analysis of clinical and biological characteristics of seven cases and review of the literature. Leuk Lymphoma. 2013;54 (4):767–77.

35. Pozzi C, D'Amico M, et al. Light chain deposition disease with renal involvement: clinical characteristics and prognostic factors. Am J Kidney Dis. 2003;42(6):1154–63.
36. Pronovost PH, Brady HR, et al. Clinical features, predictors of disease progression and results of renal transplantation in fibrillary/immunotactoid glomerulopathy. Nephrol Dial Transplant. 1996;11(5):837–42.
37. Rockx MA, Clark WF. Plasma exchange for treating cryoglobulinemia: a descriptive analysis. Transfus Apheresis Sci Official J World Apheresis Assoc Official J Eur Soc Haemapheresis. 2010;42(3):247–51.
38. Ronco PM, Alyanakian MA, et al. Light chain deposition disease: a model of glomerulosclerosis defined at the molecular level. J Am Soc Nephrol. 2001;12(7):1558–65.
39. Rosenstock JL, Markowitz GS, et al. Fibrillary and immunotactoid glomerulonephritis: distinct entities with different clinical and pathologic features. Kidney Int. 2003;63(4):1450–61.
40. Royer B, Arnulf B, et al. High dose chemotherapy in light chain or light and heavy chain deposition disease. Kidney Int. 2004;65(2):642–8.
41. Saadoun D, Pineton de Chambrun M, et al. Using rituximab plus fludarabine and cyclophosphamide as a treatment for refractory mixed cryoglobulinemia associated with lymphoma. Arthritis Care Res. 2013;65 (4):643–7.
42. Sanders PW. Mechanisms of light chain injury along the tubular nephron. J Am Soc Nephrol JASN. 2012;23(11):1777–81.
43. Sinico RA, Fornasieri A, et al. Plasma exchange in the treatment of essential mixed cryoglobulinemia nephropathy. Long-term follow up. Int J Artif Organs. 1985;8(Suppl 2):15–8.
44. Stone GC, Wall BA, et al. A vasculopathy with deposition of lambda light chain crystals. Ann Int Med. 1989;110(4):275–8.
45. Stone MJ, Bogen SA. Evidence-based focused review of management of hyperviscosity syndrome. Blood. 2012;119(10):2205–8.
46. Telio D, Shepherd J, et al. High-dose melphalan followed by auto-SCT has favorable safety and efficacy in selected patients with light chain deposition disease and light and heavy chain deposition disease. Bone Marrow Transplant. 2012;47(3):453–5.
47. Terrier B, Karras A, et al. The spectrum of type I cryoglobulinemia vasculitis: new insights based on 64 cases. Medicine. 2013;92(2):61–8.
48. Tovar N, Cibeira MT, et al. Bortezomib/dexamethasone followed by autologous stem cell transplantation as front line treatment for light-chain deposition disease. Eur J Haematol. 2012;89(4):340–4.
49. Ugai T, Tsuda K, et al. Renal Fanconi syndrome associated with monoclonal kappa free light chain in a patient with Waldenstrom macroglobulinemia. Br J Haematol. 2013;162(1):1.
50. Weichman K, Dember LM, et al. Clinical and molecular characteristics of patients with non-amyloid light chain deposition disorders, and outcome following treatment with high-dose melphalan and autologous stem cell transplantation. Bone Marrow Transplant. 2006;38(5):339–43.
51. Zand L, Kattah A, et al. C3 glomerulonephritis associated with monoclonal gammopathy: a case series. Am J Kidney Dis. 2013;62(3):506–14.

Chapter 7
Cryoglobulinemic Syndromes: Diagnosis and Management

Todd M. Zimmerman, MD

Overview

Cryoglobulinemia refers to the presence of blood proteins that precipitate at temperatures below 37 °C and subsequently redissolve when warmed. These proteins, called cryoglobulins, are composed of either monoclonal or polyclonal immunoglobulins or the combination of immunoglobulins and complement components. The composition of the cryoglobulin is dependent upon the underlying disorder, varying from lymphoproliferative disorders to autoimmune diseases and chronic infections. While the presence of cryoglobulins is most often asymptomatic, the precipitation of these proteins is associated with a variety of different clinical syndromes resulting from either the accumulation of cryoglobulins or autoimmune vasculitis. The clinical syndromes, outcome, and management vary in accordance with the underlying etiology [1]. These syndromes, which arise as a complication of these cryoglobulins, will be reviewed in this chapter.

T.M. Zimmerman, MD (✉)
Section of Hematology/Oncology, The University of Chicago, 55841 S.
Maryland Avenue, MC 2115, Chicago, IL 60637, USA
e-mail: tzimmerm@medicine.bsd.uchicago.edu

© Springer Science+Business Media New York 2017   127
T.M. Zimmerman and S.K. Kumar (eds.),
Biology and Management of Unusual Plasma Cell Dyscrasias,
DOI 10.1007/978-1-4419-6848-7_7

Classification of Cryoglobulins

The most commonly utilized classification for cryoglobulins is the Brouet classification [2] as outlined in Table 7.1. The classification is largely dependent upon determination of the clonality of the detected cryoglobulins. Type II and III cryoglobulinemia account for the majority of the cryoglobulinemic syndromes and are also referred to as mixed cryoglobulinemia; together, they account for approximately 75 % of all cases of cryoglobulinemia. This schema, while generally inclusive, does not account for all cases of cryo-globulinemia, as some cases have atypical characteristics [3, 4] and are thought potentially to represent a transition between types.

Type I—Type I cryoglobulinemia is characterized by the presence of a single monoclonal immunoglobulin, most commonly IgG or IgM and while significantly less prevalent, IgA and light chain only cryoglobulins have been reported. The underlying cause of Type I cryoglobulinemia is a monoclonal expansion of B cells, most often an underlying antibody-producing lymphoproliferative disorders. In a large series of patients with Type I cryoglobulinemia [5], monoclonal gammopathy of unknown significance was the most common diagnosis, accounting for 44 % of the cases and overt malignancies accounted for the remaining cases. Of those patients with a malignancy, Waldenstrom's macroglobulinemia and multiple myeloma accounted for 70 % of the cases.

Table 7.1 Brouet classification for cryoglobulinemia

Class	
Cryoglobulin component	Common underlying conditions
Type I	
Monoclonal immunoglobulin	Lymphoproliferative disorders
Mixed cryoglobulinemias	
Type II	
Monoclonal component and polyclonal immunoglobulin	Hepatitis C infection
Type III	
No monoclonal present	Autoimmune disorders

Type II—Type II cryoglobulinemia is mixture of polyclonal immunoglobulins in association with a monoclonal rheumatoid factor. These cases are frequently associated with persistent viral infections, most commonly hepatitis C, but human immunodeficiency viruses and Epstein–Barr have also been reported [6].

Type III—Type III cryoglobulins consist of both polyclonal immunoglobulins and polyclonal rheumatoid factors. These are frequently associated with connective tissue disease, although infections with hepatitis C still account for a significant percentage of the cases.

Prevalence, Etiology, and Pathogenesis

Prevalence

The presence of small amounts of cryoglobulin is not necessarily a sign of disease as minute levels of cryoglobulin have been detected in many healthy people, and polyclonal cryoglobulins have transiently been detected during some viral and bacterial infection [7]. The overall incidence of cryoglobulinemia has not been well established as the prevalence of viral infections can vary considerably in different populations. The incidence of detectable cryoglobulin has been reported in 15–20 % of patients with HIV, 15–25 % of patients with autoimmune disorders and 40–65 % of patients with hepatitis C [8–10]. While the presence of asymptomatic cryoglobulinemia remains poorly defined, symptomatic cryoglobulinemia is considered a relatively rare condition estimated at ten per million people [11]. It also appears to be more common in women than men with a peak between the ages of 45 and 65 years [12, 13].

Etiology and Pathogenesis

Type I—Type I cryoglobulinemic states are brought on by the monoclonal immunoglobulin which is produced by the underlying lymphoproliferative process. Outside of the manifestations of the underlying malignancy, there are several unique mechanisms by which Type I cryoglobulinemia can manifest clinical symptoms. The monoclonal immunoglobulin can itself cause hyperviscosity with its associated clinical symptomatology, and the cold induced precipitates physically obstruct small to medium sized vessel, thereby mediating an inflammatory vasculitis.

Type II and III—Although lymphoproliferative disorders have been associated with type II and III cryoglobulinemic syndromes, the mixed cryoglobulinemic states are most often resultant from chronic viral infections and chronic inflammatory states including connective tissue disorders [14]. Many of these clinical syndromes arise from an expansion of cryoglobulinemic B cells [15], and the most intensely studied of these states is in the setting of patients with hepatitis C infections.

Clinical Manifestations

Although cryoglobulinemia simply refers to the presence of the cryoglobulin, the clinical manifestations that result are primarily caused by small to medium vessel vasculitis from the cryoglobulin-containing immune complexes. Most investigators have used the terms cryoglobulinemic syndrome or cryoglobulin vasculitis to describe the presence of the clinical manifestations in the presence of a cryoglobulin, as opposed to the asymptomatic presence of a cryoglobulin without clinical manifestations.

Type I—The clinical spectrum of Type I cryoglobulinemia differs from the mixed cryoglobulinemias, Type II and III. In addition, much of the symptomatology in patients with Type I cryoglobulinemia are related to the underlying malignancy and may include symptomatic anemia, constitutional symptoms, and skeletal complications. Other common clinical manifestations of Type I cryoglobulinemia are related to hyperviscosity or thrombosis and include livedo reticularis, purpura, Raynaud's phenomenon, digital ischemia, and thrombosis which in severe cases can progress to gangrene [16]. Neurologic syndromes related to hyperviscosity are often exhibited as well, manifesting as visual changes, epistaxis, headache, and in severe cases, stroke or coma [17]. These symptoms are most commonly noted in patients with Waldenstrom's macroglobulinemia and multiple myeloma.

In a recent series of 64 patients with symptomatic cryoglobulinemia [18], almost 80 % of patients presented with severe systemic vasculitis which included extensive cutaneous ulcerations, peripheral neuropathy, and glomerulonephritis. Overall, dermatologic features were the most common features, including purpura, acrocyanosis, skin necrosis, skin ulcers, and livedo reticularis. Systemic manifestations included peripheral neuropathy, and renal and joint involvement.

Type II and III—The mixed cryoglobulinemias (Type II and III) commonly cause systemic and constitutional symptoms including arthralgias, fatigue, peripheral neuropathy, and palpable purpura which in some cases can lead to cutaneous ulcerations. Concurrent with the clinical manifestations of the Type II and III cryoglobulinemia, the underlying etiologic condition including infectious process or autoimmune disorders complicates the clinical picture with additional symptoms related to the infection or autoimmune disorder. An underlying etiology for the cryoglobulinemia can be identified for the vast majority of patients, but if a cause cannot be identified, it is classified as essential cryoglobulinemia.

The classic clinical feature of mixed cryoglobulinemia is Meltzer's triad, consisting of palpable purpura, arthralgia, and weakness, but this triad is seen in as few as 25–30 % of patients [19, 20]. Cutaneous manifestations occur in most patients with mixed cryoglobulinemia and can precede other systemic manifestations by years [21]. Musculoskeletal complaints including myalgias and arthralgias are common, but frank arthritis is uncommon [22]. Finally, peripheral neuropathy afflicts a high number of patients with mixed cryoglobulinemia [23], much higher than seen with Type I cryoglobulinemia. Other organ involvement including subclinical pulmonary involvement and renal disease is most commonly associated with immune complex disease [24, 25].

Laboratory Evaluation

The initial diagnostic approach to a patient with suspected cryo-globulinemia should focus on two features. First, identification and characterization of the cryoglobulin are crucial for establishing the diagnosis but can help guide the second goal of the evaluation, the identification and characterization of the causative disorder, which is crucial for long-term management and control of the disease.

Cryoglobulin

The first step toward the evaluation of a patient with suspected cryoglobulinemia is the identification and characterization of the cryoglobulin [26]. If a cryoglobulin is suspected, a cryocrit should be requested for the detection and quantification of the cryoglob-ulin. The value which is typically reported as percentage and the final level may take several days to completely precipitate. If a cryoglobulin is identified, the precipitate can be dissolved upon warming. The redissolved cryoglobulin can be further character-ized with immune electrophoresis or other immunologic assays so as to help guide the evaluation of the underlying etiology. If the clinical suspicion remains high and the cryocrit is negative, repeat testing should be performed after consultation with the laboratory in order to ensure appropriate handling of the specimen. Furthermore, as it may take several days for the full precipitation of the cryoglobulin, especially for Type III cryoglobulinemia, await-ing the final analysis is important to rule out the presence of a cryoglobulin.

SPEP/Immunofixation

Of particular importance for patients with Type I Cryoglobulinemia is the detection and characterization of monoclonal immunoglob-ulin which is helpful for the diagnosis and eventual management of the underlying malignancy. In addition to the monoclonal immunoglobulin, mild to moderate polyclonal expansion of immunoglobulins can be seen in all types of cryoglobulinemia and is indicative of the inflammatory state. Furthermore, classical markers of inflammation, including elevation of erythrocyte sedimentation rate (ESR) and C-reactive protein, are frequently seen and can be supportive of the diagnosis. When symptomatic hyperviscosity is suspected, a serum viscosity should be ordered; symptoms are usually not seen unless the serum viscosity exceeds 4.0 centipoise [27].

Complement/Autoantibodies

Decreased serum complement levels are indicators of ongoing consumption by the precipitation process and are useful for the diagnosis and monitoring the eventual response to therapy. Type I cryoglobulinemia less commonly results in suppression of complement levels which is most often noted in patients with mixed cryoglobulinemia. The most common laboratory pattern is a decrease in total hemolytic complement (CH50) as well as early complement proteins including C1q, C2, and C4 [28, 29].

Infectious Workup

Of particular importance in patients with mixed cryoglobulinemia, a careful evaluation for underlying etiology is crucial. As ongoing viral infections, particularly hepatitis C, is the most common cause of mixed cryoglobulinemia, serologic evaluation for viral hepatitis should be performed but assessment of other viral infections including Epstein–Barr virus and HIV should be included in the workup of these patients [30, 31].

Pathologic Findings

Cutaneous

Cutaneous manifestations of cryoglobulinemic vasculitis may be manifested by palpable purpura, petechia, or even ulcers. Skin lesions associated with Type I cryoglobulins are most often non-inflammatory thrombotic lesions while skin lesion from mixed cryoglobulins frequently reveal leukocytoclastic vasculitis and less commonly inflammatory or non-inflammatory purpura [32]. Direct immunofluorescence of acute lesions frequently reveals deposits of IgG, IgM, or C3 complement [33].

Peripheral Nerve

Peripheral nerve involvement, which is frequently asymptomatic, affects a high number of patients with mixed cryoglobulinemia and is less commonly exhibited in patients with Type I cryoglobulinemia. Some studies have demonstrated EMG and NCV abnormalities in up to 80 % of patients, but symptomatic in a much smaller number of patients [34, 35]. Microscopic evaluations of the lesions typically demonstrate vasculitis and affected nerves demonstrate axonal degeneration.

Renal

Renal involvement is frequently encountered in patients with cryoglobulinemia, and approximately 30 % of patients have some degree of renal impairment at diagnosis [36]. Renal biopsy typically demonstrates membranoproliferative glomerulonephritis [37]. Hypertension is common among patients with membranoproliferative glomerulonephritis and cryoglobulinemia and frequently is the presenting manifestation for many patients.

Bone Marrow

The bone marrow biopsy in patients with Type I cryoglobulinemia will often reveal the presence of the underlying lymphoproliferative disorder or plasma cell dyscrasia. Commonly associated conditions include monoclonal gammopathy of unknown significance, multiple myeloma, and Waldenstrom's macroglobulinemia. The morphologic and genetic information obtained from the bone marrow biopsy is crucial for the diagnosis and therapeutic approach. The bone marrow findings in patients with mixed cryoglobulinemia have not been well described and should only be done when the clinical situation dictates.

Diagnosis and Differential

The diagnosis of symptomatic cryoglobulinemia is frequently made when a patient presents with symptoms typically seen with vasculitic involvement of the involved organs, primarily the skin and kidneys. With suspected cryoglobulinemia, repeat testing for the presence of the cryoglobulin should be pursued if the initial test was negative since false negatives are not uncommon. Furthermore, the cryoglobulin, particularly in patients with Type III cryoglobulinemia, may take several days to precipitate. Prior to ordering, a discussion of the testing with the phlebotomist and performing laboratory can help ensure the proper handling on the specimen if repeat testing is requested. Additional testing as described earlier, including serum chemistries, serum electrophoresis, complement levels, and rheumatologic evaluation, acute phase reactants, and infectious serologies should be performed. Tissue biopsy of suspected involved organs should also be performed to determine the extent of involvement. A preliminary international classification system has been developed and is outlined in Table 7.2 [38].

The differential diagnosis of cryoglobulinemic vasculitis includes other vasculitis syndromes that affect small to medium sized vessels, including vasculitides associated with drug hypersensitivity and those associated with autoimmune disorders.

Table 7.2 Preliminary classification for the diagnosis of cryoglobulinemic vasculitis

Item 1:	Subjective symptoms
Positive answer to at least two of the questions	
A.	Do you remember one or more episodes of small red spots on your skin, particularly involving the lower limbs?
B.	Have you ever had red spots on your lower extremities which leave a brownish color after their disappearance?
C.	Has a doctor ever told you that you have viral hepatitis?
Item 2:	**Objective Symptoms (present or past)**
Presence of at least three of the following:	
A.	Constitutional symptoms (fatigue, fever, fibromyalgia)
B.	Articular involvement (arthralgias, arthritis)
C.	Vascular involvement (purpura, skin ulcers, necrotizing vasculitis, hyperviscosity syndrome, Raynaud phenomenon)
D.	Neurologic involvement (peripheral neuropathy, cranial nerve involvement, CNS involvement)
Item 3:	**Laboratory abnormalities**
Presence at the time of the diagnosis of at least two of the following:	
A.	Low serum C4 levels
B.	Positive serum rheumatoid factor
C.	Positive serum M component

Criteria fulfillment: at least two of the three items in a patient with cryoglobulinemia (serum cryoglobulins detected at least two times during an interval of at least 12 weeks)

Disorders that mimic vasculitis may also be confused infectious as well as thrombotic and embolic disorders.

Clinical Management

The management of patients with cryoglobulinemia is dependent upon the underlying disorder and the severity of the syndrome. Addressing the complications of the cryoglobulinemia is absolutely crucial to the management of patients with cryoglobulinemia.

These complications often require emergent therapy and should be addressed prior to the management of the underlying condition. For patients presenting with symptomatic hyperviscosity, urgent plasmapheresis is required to remove the cryoglobulin. While plasmapheresis will help alleviate the signs and symptoms of hyperviscosity, the effects are temporary and additional therapy to manage the underlying condition is required to prevent recurrence of the symptoms and complications.

Management of Type I

In patients with Type I cryoglobulinemia, the therapy should target the underlying lymphoproliferative disorder. In a series of sixty-four patients with Type I cryoglobulinemia and vasculitis [39], fifty-six received at least one course of treatment. The vast majority of patients received corticosteroids and in patients with underlying MGUS, additional therapy with plasmapheresis, immunosuppressant agents, or rituximab was also required in a significant portion of the patients. For patients with more overt malignancies, such as multiple myeloma or Waldenstrom's macroglobulinemia, treatment of the malignancy helps provide longer term control.

Management of Mixed CG

In contrast to Type I cryoglobulinemia, the mixed cryoglobulinemias are associated with a number of different underlying conditions varying from viral infections to autoimmune disorders and malignancies. If a known cause of the cryoglobulin cannot be identified, it is termed essential cryoglobulinemia. The main cause of mixed cryoglobulinemia is persistent infections, of which hepatitis C infections account for 90 % of all cases [40].

Antiviral therapy should be considered for all patients with HCV, and the introduction of the new agents including the protease inhibitors has changed the outcomes for patients with mixed cryoglobulinemia related to hepatitis C infections [41]. The use of non-interferon-containing regimens has improved tolerability of hepatitis C therapy, and all patients diagnosed with such an infection should be referred to an appropriate specialist in the field. The most promising non-antiviral therapy for patients with mixed CG has been B-cell depletion therapy with rituximab. In two prospective trials of patients with mixed CG and hepatitis C infections, the addition of rituximab to standard antiviral therapy improved the outcomes for patients compare to patients treated with antiviral therapy alone [42, 43].

For patients with non-infectious mixed CG, the most common cause is autoimmune disorders yet in about half of the cases, no etiology has been identified. The therapeutic approach to non-infectious mixed CG is focused on the use of immunosuppressive agents which suppress B-cell clonal expansion similar to strategies of other vasculitides including azathioprine, glucocorticoids, and cytotoxic chemotherapy agents such as cyclophosphamide [44]. Likewise, the addition of rituximab to corticosteroid therapy resulted in improved outcomes, and in another meta-analysis, rituximab was superior to other agents including alkylating agents and other immunosuppressive agents [45]. While the rate of severe infection was higher in those patients receiving rituximab, the mortality was not higher.

Conclusion

The cryoglobulinemia syndromes consist of a conglomerate of syndromes in which a cryoglobulin, made up of immunoglobulin and complement component precipitates upon cooling. While the majority of the patients with a cryoglobulin are asymptomatic, the clinical syndrome that is often resultant from the cryoglobulin requires a thorough understanding of the disease, a careful diagnosis, and thoughtful management. The Brouet classification uses the clonality of the cryoglobulin to define the subtype, and the clinical manifestations vary upon the type of cryoglobulinemia Type I versus mixed cryoglobulinemias (Type II or III). Likewise, the management is contingent upon the underlying condition that gave rise to the cryoglobulin. Immediate management of the organ-specific complications is necessary if required, but management of the underlying condition, if identified, is crucial to long-term control. In Type I cryoglobulinemia, treatment of the underlying lymphoproliferative disorder remains the focus of the primary management, while with the mixed cryoglobulinemia, the management is dependent upon treating the infectious or non-infectious etiology. For patients with infectious mixed cryoglobulinemia, the combination of antiviral therapy and rituximab appears to result in improved outcomes while those patients with non-infectious, or essential CG, the combination of corticosteroids and rituximab should be considered.

References

1. Ramos-Casals M, Stone JH, Cid MC, Bosch X. The cryoglobulinaemias. Lancet. 2012;379(9813):348–60.
2. Brouet JC, Clauvel JP, Danon F, Klein M, Seligmann M. Biologic and clinical significance of cryoglobulins. A report of 86 cases. Am J Med. 1974;57(5):775–88.
3. Musset L, Diemert MC, Taibi F, et al. Characterization of cryoglobulins by immunoblotting. Clin Chem. 1992;38:798.
4. Tissot JD, Schifferli JA, Hochstrasser DF, et al. Two-dimensional polyacrylamide gel electrophoresis analysis of cryoglobulins and identification of an IgM-associated peptide. J Immunol Methods. 1994;173:63.
5. Terrier B, Karras A, Kahn JE, et al. The spectrum of type I cryoglobulinemia vasculitis: new insights based on 64 cases. Medicine. 2013;92:61–8.
6. Fabris P, Tositti G, Giordani MT, et al. Prevalence and clinical significance of circulating cryoglobulins in HIV-positive patients with and without co-infection with hepatitis C virus. J Med Virol. 2003;69:339.
7. Sargur R, White P, Egner W. Cryoglobulin evaluation: best practice? Ann Clin Biochem. 2010;47:8–16.
8. Bonnet F, Pineau JJ, Taupin JL, et al. Prevalence of cryoglobulinemia and serological markers of autoimmunity in human immunodeficiency virus infected individuals: a cross-sectional study of 97 patients. J Rheumatol. 2003;30:2005.
9. García-Carrasco M, Ramos-Casals M, Cervera R, et al. Cryoglobulinemia in systemic lupus erythematosus: prevalence and clinical characteristics in a series of 122 patients. Semin Arthritis Rheum. 2001;30:366.
10. Cicardi M, Cesana B, Del Ninno E, et al. Prevalence and risk factors for the presence of serum cryoglobulins in patients with chronic hepatitis C. J Viral Hepat. 2000;7:138.

11. Gorevic PD, Kassab HJ, Levo Y, et al. Mixed cryoglobulinemia: clinical aspects and long-term follow-up of 40 patients. Am J Med. 1980;69:287.

12. Saadoun D, Sellam J, Ghillani-Dalbin P, et al. Increased risks of lymphoma and death among patients with non-hepatitis C virus-related mixed cryoglobulinemia. Arch Intern Med. 2006;166:2101.

13. Ferri C, Zignego AL, Pileri SA. Cryoglobulins. J Clin Pathol. 2002;55:4–13.

14. Terrier B, Cacoub P. Cryoglobulinemic vasculitis: an update. Curr Opin Rheumatol. 2013;25:10.

15. De Re V, De Vita S, Sansonno D, et al. Type II mixed cryoglobulinaemia as an oligo rather than a mono B-cell disorder: evidence from GeneScan and MALDI-TOF analyses. Rheumatology (Oxford). 2006;45:685.

16. Cohen SJ, Pittelkow MR, Su WP. Cutaneous manifestations of cryoglobulinemia: clinical and histopathologic study of seventy-two patients. J Am Acad Dermatol. 1991;25:21.

17. Gertz MA, Kyle RA. Hyperviscosity syndrome. J Intensive Care Med. 1995;10(3):128–41.

18. Terrier B, Karras A, Kahn JE, et al. The spectrum of type I cryoglobulinemia vasculitis: new insights based on 64 cases. Medicine (Baltimore). 2013;92:61–8.

19. Meltzer M, Franklin EC. Cryoglobulinemia—a study of twenty-nine patients. I. IgG and IgM cryoglobulins and factors affecting cryoprecipitability. Am J Med. 1966;40:828.

20. Montagnino G. Reappraisal of the clinical expression of mixed cryoglobulinemia. Springer Semin Immunopathol. 1988;10:1.

21. Nash JW, Ross P Jr, Neil Crowson A, et al. The histopathologic spectrum of cryofibrinogenemia in four anatomic sites. Skin, lung, muscle, and kidney. Am J Clin Pathol. 2003;119:114.

22. Weinberger A, Berliner S, Pinkhas J. Articular manifestations of essential cryoglobulinemia. Semin Arthritis Rheum. 1981;10:224.

23. Gemignani F, Pavesi G, Fiocchi A, et al. Peripheral neuropathy in essential mixed cryoglobulinaemia. J Neurol Neurosurg Psychiatry. 1992;55:116.

24. Viegi G, Fornai E, Ferri C, et al. Lung function in essential mixed cryoglobulinemia: a short-term follow-up. Clin Rheumatol. 1989;8:331.

25. Beddhu S, Bastacky S, Johnson JP. The clinical and morphologic spectrum of renal cryoglobulinemia. Medicine (Baltimore). 2002;81:398.

26. Vermeersch P, Gijbels K, Mariën G, et al. A critical appraisal of current practice in the detection, analysis, and reporting of cryoglobulins. Clin Chem. 2008;54:39.

27. Stone MJ, Bogen SA. Evidence-based focused review of management of hyperviscosity syndrome. Blood. 2012;119:2205–8.

28. Monti G, Galli M, Invernizzi F, et al. Cryoglobulinaemias: a multi-centre study of the early clinical and laboratory manifestations of primary and secondary disease. GISC. Italian Group for the study of cryoglobulinaemias. QJM. 1995;88:115.

29. Tarantino A, Anelli A, Costantino A, et al. Serum complement pattern in essential mixed cryoglobulinaemia. Clin Exp Immunol. 1978;32:77.

30. Agnello V, Chung RT, Kaplan LM. A role for hepatitis C virus infection in type II cryoglobulinemia. N Engl J Med. 1992;327:1490.
31. Misiani R, Bellavita P, Fenili D, et al. Hepatitis C virus infection in patients with essential mixed cryoglobulinemia. Ann Intern Med. 1992;117:573.
32. Gorevic PD, Kassab HJ, Levo Y, et al. Mixed cryoglobulinemia: clinical aspects and long-term follow-up of 40 patients. Am J Med. 1980;69:287.
33. Cohen SJ, Pittelkow MR, Su WP. Cutaneous manifestations of cryoglobulinemia: clinical and histopathologic study of seventy-two patients. J Am Acad Dermatol. 1991;25:21.
34. Ferri C, La Civita L, Cirafisi C, et al. Peripheral neuropathy in mixed cryoglobulinemia: clinical and electrophysiologic investigations. J Rheumatol. 1992;19:889.
35. Gemignani F, Pavesi G, Fiocchi A, et al. Peripheral neuropathy in essential mixed cryoglobulinaemia. J Neurol Neurosurg Psychiatry. 1992;55:116.
36. Tarantino A, De Vecchi A, Montagnino G, et al. Renal disease in essential mixed cryoglobulinaemia. Long-term follow-up of 44 patients. Q J Med. 1981;50:1.
37. Schena FP. Survey of the Italian registry of renal biopsies. Frequency of the renal diseases for 7 consecutive years. The Italian Group of renal immunopathology. Nephrol Dial Transplant. 1997;12:418.
38. De Vita S, Soldano F, Isola M, et al. Preliminary classification criteria for the cryoglobulinaemic vasculitis. Ann Rheum Dis. 2011;70:1183–90.
39. Terrier B1, Karras A, Kahn JE, Le Guenno G, Marie I, Benarous L, Lacraz A, Diot E, Hermine O, de Saint-Martin L, Cathébras P, Leblond V, Modiano P, Léger JM, Mariette X, Senet P, Plaisier E, Saadoun D, Cacoub P. The spectrum of type I cryoglobulinemia vasculitis: new insights based on 64 cases. Medicine (Baltimore). 2013;92(2):61–8.
40. Ramos-Casals M, Stone JH, Cid MC, Bosch X. The cryoglobulinaemias. Lancet. 2012;379:348.
41. Kohli A, Shaffer A, Sherman A, Kottilil S. Treatment of hepatitis C. A systematic review. JAMA. 2014;312:631.
42. Sneller MC, Hu Z, Langford CA. A randomized controlled trial of rituximab following failure of antiviral therapy for hepatitis C virus-associated cryoglobulinemic vasculitis. Arthritis Rheum. 2012;64 (835–42):35.
43. De Vita S, Quartuccio L, Isola M, et al. A randomized controlled trial of rituximab for the treatment of severe cryoglobulinemic vasculitis. Arthritis Rheum. 2012;64:843–53.
44. Terrier B, Krastinova E, Marie I, et al. Management of noninfectious mixed cryoglobulinemia vasculitis: data from 242 cases included in the CryoVas survey. Blood. 2012;119:5996–6004.
45. Terrier B, Launay D, Kaplanski G, et al. Safety and efficacy of rituximab in nonviral cryoglobulinemia vasculitis: data from the French Autoimmunity and Rituximab registry. Arthritis Care Res (Hoboken). 2010;62:1787–95.

Chapter 8
Idiopathic Systemic Capillary Leak Syndrome (Clarkson Disease)

Prashant Kapoor, MD

Introduction

Idiopathic systemic capillary leak syndrome (SCLS) or Clarkson disease is an exceedingly rare, but potentially fatal disorder related to microvascular hyperpermeability. Massive leakage of intravascular fluids and macromolecules manifests clinically as stereotypical "attacks" or "flares" of transient, but profound hypotension and generalized edema [1]. During an acute episode, hemoconcentration and hypoalbuminemia develop as a result of capillary hyperpermeability. However, during the asymptomatic periods, inbetween the attacks, serum monoclonal protein and elevated plasma vascular endothelial growth factor (VEGF) may be the only laboratory abnormalities pointing toward SCLS [2–4].

It can be challenging to give a unifying diagnosis of idiopathic SCLS to a patient presenting with a perplexing and rapidly progressive symptomatology and non-specific laboratory abnormalities. As such, the disorder is often misdiagnosed upon initial presentation,

P. Kapoor, MD (✉)
Division of Hematology, Department of Medicine, Mayo Clinic,
200 First Street SW, Rochester, MN 55905, USA
e-mail: kapoor.prashant@mayo.edu

© Springer Science+Business Media New York 2017   143
T.M. Zimmerman and S.K. Kumar (eds.),
Biology and Management of Unusual Plasma Cell Dyscrasias,
DOI 10.1007/978-1-4419-6848-7_8

and the true incidence of SCLS remains unknown. Notably, during the last two decades, the number of published cases has surged, likely a reflection of increased awareness of this enigmatic disease among clinicians [5, 6]. Several new cases have been reported from all over the world since the initial reports of SCLS from the United States and Europe [7–10].

History

The eponym, Clarkson syndrome, traces its roots to a case described in 1960 by Bayard Clarkson and colleagues, of a young female with persistent paraproteinemia who ultimately succumbed to a cyclical illness characterized by episodes of low grade fevers, anasarca, hypovolemic shock, hypoalbuminemia, and elevated hematocrit [11]. In 1962, another case with similar features involving a 29-year-old man with flares of anasarca, urticaria, fever, and malaise in the background of increased serum gamma globulins, splenomegaly, and marked eosinophilia (50–70 %) was published [12]. However, unlike the index case, hypotension was conspicuously absent. This case of episodic angioedema with eosinophilia went on to be later recognized as Gleich's syndrome [13, 14].

Subsequently, in 1963, Weinbren suggested the term "spontaneous periodic edema" instead of "cyclical edema" for the cluster of recurrent symptoms similar to those originally described by Clarkson et al. that would spontaneously develop in a 45-year-old Englishman with sporadic bouts of edema [15]. Four years later, in 1967, Melvin Horwith who had described the index case with Clarkson reported another fatal case of hypovolemic shock of unknown etiology. The postmortem study revealed diffuse interstitial edema, pulmonary edema, and serous effusions [16]. Over the course of the next two decades, only 20 more accounts appeared in the medical literature, attesting to the rarity of this sporadic disorder [17, 18].

In 1992 and 1999, two small case series from Mayo Clinic reported on the efficacy of terbutaline and aminophylline in idiopathic SCLS [19, 20]. In 1997, a larger, multicenter, retrospective, French study outlined the course of SCLS and evaluated the efficacy of the available therapies in a cohort of 13 patients [21]. By the year 2006, approximately one hundred cases of idiopathic SCLS had been reported worldwide. More recently, two larger studies, one from Mayo Clinic and the other from a European registry, reported on the clinical experience with 25 and 28 patients with SCLS, respectively, shedding light on the nuances in the diagnosis and management of idiopathic SCLS [22, 23]. Regardless, there remains a paucity of high-level evidence and even though single case reports in various clinical settings continue to be a major source of clinical information currently, caution should be exercised in interpreting anecdotal reports, particularly with regard to the management.

Definition and Pathogenesis

The criteria for the diagnosis of SCLS include documentation of recurrent characteristic attacks of (1) hypotension, (2) elevated hematocrit, (3) peripheral edema, and (4) hypoalbuminemia in the absence of albuminuria [22]. Importantly, resolution of the attacks is accompanied with the normalization of hematocrit and albumin levels. Monoclonal gammopathy is not a mandatory criterion, albeit its presence in the appropriate clinical setting serves as a useful diagnostic clue [22]. Clinically relevant disease-related information is available at the National Organization of Rare Disorders Web site as well as a patient-support Web site, www.rareshare.org.

The molecular events that trigger the episodic vascular hyper-permeability are unknown, and the pathogenesis of SCLS remains indeterminate [24]. Immune dysregulation, cytokines, leukotrienes, VEGF, and complement system have been implicated. Interleukin-2 receptor-positive peripheral blood mononuclear cell counts can increase substantially during periods of hyperperme-ability [25]. Proteins with weights up to 900 kilodaltons can extravasate. Ultrastructural studies have revealed endothelial apoptosis including endothelial microvesicular body and bleb formation during attacks, suggesting disruption of the microvas-culature [26]. Sera of patients with SCLS have been found to possess endothelial cell damaging properties. This mechanism appears to be distinct from other edema-associated conditions, including anaphylaxis in which the endothelial shape changes and widening of intercellular gaps rather than apoptosis are associated with swelling [3, 24].

A majority (76–90 %) of patients with SCLS has concurrent evidence of monoclonal gammopathy; a notable proportion compared to the 3 percent incidence of monoclonal gammopathy of undetermined significance (MGUS) in the general population over 50 years of age [22, 23]. A few accounts of SCLS with other plasma cell disorders, including plasma cell leukemia, multiple myeloma, and amyloidosis have been published [4, 5, 8, 22, 23, 27, 28]. However, a direct monoclonal protein-mediated vascular injury has never been proven [26, 29]. Moreover, cytotoxicity has not been observed on exposure of the cultured endothelial cells to the purified monoclonal protein [29]. It has been hypothesized that the monoclonal protein could potentially inhibit a factor integral for maintaining the endothelial barrier function [3].

Two studies which reported on increase in interleukin-6 and tumor necrosis factor-alpha levels in the sera of SCLS patients hinted on the possibility of the systemic inflammatory response. However, recent studies have counteracted this observation highlighting the lack of a prominent role of inflammation in SCLS. In contradistinction, inflammation plays a dominant role in sepsis associated with the vascular leak [24]. Laboratory evidence suggests that high baseline, as well as intra-attack levels of plasma VEGF (previously called vascular permeability factor) and angiopoietin-2 (Ang 2), is instrumental in inducing capillary hyperpermeability [3]. However, much remains to be clarified regarding the molecular processes that induce promoters of enhanced vascular permeability. Blood samples of 20 patients with acute SCLS and 3 patients with chronic SCLS were collected to perform experiments studying the effects of SCLS sera on human microvascular endothelial cells (HMVECs). Upon application of the sera obtained from patients at the onset of an attack (episodic sera), HMVECs demonstrated interendothelial junction disruption, retraction, and hyperpermeability (through internalization of the junctional protein VE cadherin), but not apoptosis. These effects on HMVEC were, however, not recapitulated when the sera obtained during remission or the IgG isolated from episodic sera were utilized. Serum VEGF and Ang 2 levels were found to be substantially elevated during acute episodes compared to quiescent phases. Interestingly, the elevated VEGF levels at onset have been shown to precipitously decline during the course of an attack and return to baseline prior to the onset of the "post-leak" phase. Pretreatment with intravenous immunoglobulin and anti-Ang 2, but not anti-VEGF antibody, bevacizumab, demonstrated a protective effect on the capillary permeability [3].

Correlating with the mechanistic studies of SCLS sera outlined above, the NIH group recently reported the preliminary findings of genomewide single nucleotide polymorphism (SNP) analysis in 12 patients with SCLS, the first nine of whom also underwent whole-exome sequencing. Interestingly, SNPs were identified in the genes with potential role in endothelial barrier function or capillary permeability. Additionally, SNPs in genes related to clonal plasma cell expansion were discovered [30].

Epidemiology

Middle aged adults of Caucasian race are more likely to be affected by idiopathic SCLS, but a wide variation in the age at presentation has been observed. The disorder has also been reported in both Asians and Blacks [5]. The largest case series to date from a European registry attempts to shed light on the epidemiological aspects, laboratory findings, and management [23]. In this study, 28 consecutive patients with SCLS from 34 medical centers in 5 countries were prospectively monitored over 13 years. The median age at onset of attacks was 49 years (range: 5–78 years) and at diagnosis was 53. Only two patients were Black. The median frequency of attacks per patient was 4.5 attacks (range, 1–59), including two severe attacks per patient. No gender preponderance was noted in the Mayo Clinic or the European study [22, 23]. However, the European registry study demonstrated that the first manifestation of SCLS occurs more than a decade later in men [23].

A single case of familial SCLS has been reported in a Jewish family [31], and additionally, the appearance of this syndrome in a 17-day-old newborn in the Mayo Clinic series raises the possibility of intrauterine transfer of soluble mediators or an inherited disorder [22].

Clinical Symptoms, Signs, and Diagnostic Challenges

Massive third-spacing of fluids and protein leakage as a consequence of endothelial barrier dysfunction leads to various clinical manifestations. The attacks classically start spontaneously, rapidly progress within a few hours and resolve within 1–4 days. Remobilization of fluids back into the intravascular compartment occurs just as spontaneously as the flares arise, leading to resolution of symptoms and diuresis [24].

Attacks often appear to be unprovoked. Triggers for attacks include upper respiratory tract infection (74 %); physical strain and nearly a quarter of female patients have experienced intramenstruation flares [22].

Although non-specific, prodromal symptoms (Fig. 8.1) of profound fatigue (88 %), presyncope/ lightheadedness (76 %), myalgias or flu-like symptoms (56 %), throat irritation (32 %), reduced urinary output (28 %), or rarely mood changes (4 %) have been observed. While such symptoms may vary among patients, for an individual patient, the prodromal symptoms prior to a flare are generally similar, and if recognized early, can alert a patient to see prompt medical attention [22].

A serotypical "flare" or an "attack" is characterized by a tetrad of vascular collapse or hypotension, generalized edema, hemoconcentration, and hypoalbuminemia. The edema characteristically worsens on initial intravenous fluid resuscitation (Fig. 8.1) [22]. In the Mayo Clinic series, 76 % of patients presented with generalized or localized body ache, 64 % with facial edema, and over one-half with dyspnea. Nearly a third of patients had nausea and/or vomiting. Loss of consciousness and/or weight gain was also noted in approximately a third of patients [22].

Polydipsia with salt craving, headache, diaphoresis, fever, rhinorrhea, hoarseness, arthralgia, lacrimation, pruritus, flushing, dysphagia, and jaw claudication are some of the other features that can be observed during a flare [22, 23].

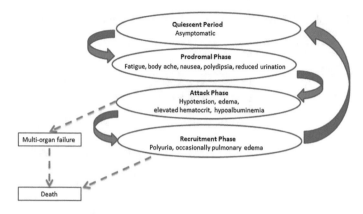

Fig. 8.1 Different phases of idiopathic systemic capillary leak syndrome

Timely and accurate diagnosis of SCLS can be challenging, particularly with the first episode. It is important to consider this rare entity in any individual presenting with edema and shock. In the Mayo Clinic study, 25 patients evaluated over a 27-year period fulfilled all the diagnostic criteria for SCLS. The series highlighted the delay in diagnosis as suggested by the median time of 1.13 years (range: 0–32) between the onset of symptoms and definitive diagnosis. A unifying diagnosis was made more than five years after onset of symptoms in 12 % of the patients in that series. In the European study, the median delay in diagnosis was 7 months (range, 0–110 months) [22, 23]. Unless the first attack is fatal, classic clinical course entails recurrence of symptoms, with substantially varying frequency or severity of attacks among patients. Considerable delay in the diagnosis, in part, results from the lack of specific symptoms and distinct findings that would be attributable to this diagnosis of exclusion. Patients with SCLS are often initially misdiagnosed as other conditions with overlapping features (Table 8.1).

During the quiescent period inbetween the attacks, the physical examination is typically unremarkable, except in patients with chronic SCLS who exhibit long-standing generalized edema with serous (pleural and pericardial) effusions [32].

All patients demonstrate hemoconcentration during an attack. In the Mayo series, the median absolute increase in hematocrit was

Table 8.1 Differential diagnoses of idiopathic systemic capillary leak syndrome

Alternative diagnosis	Disease features
Secondary SCLS [62–67]	Hypotension, edema, presence of inciting factors (alpha- and beta-interferon, acitretin, gemcitabine, interleukin-2, denileukin diftitox and filgrastim, hepatitis C infection, post-stem cell transplantation, and malignancies
Polycythemia vera [68]	Erythrocytosis, thrombocytosis, leukocytosis, DVT, low erythropoietin levels, JAK 2V617F mutation
Gleich's syndrome [13]	Cyclic edema, urticaria, eosinophilia, elevated IgM
Carcinoid syndrome	Flushing, hypotension, elevated 5HT3, and its metabolites
Mastocytosis	Elevated tryptase and urticaria pigmentosa
Nephrotic syndrome	Anasarca, proteinuria, and hypoalbuminemia
Sepsis	Hypotension, edema, fever, and leucocytosis
Acute gastroenteritis	Nausea, vomiting, and abdominal pain
Congestive heart failure	Edema, hypotension, and dyspnea
Toxic shock syndrome	Hypotension, leucocytosis, and desquamatory rash
Hereditary angioedema	Low C1 esterase inhibitor or function
AL amyloidosis	Edema, monoclonal protein, diarrhea, and proteinuria
Pancreatitis	Nausea, vomiting, abdominal pain, and elevated pancreatic enzymes
Adrenal insufficiency	Hypotension, abdominal pain, and hyponatremia
POEMS syndrome [69]	**P**olyneuropathy, **O**rganomegaly, **E**ndocrinopathy, **M**onoclonal gammopathy, **S**kin changes, polycythemia, edema, elevated VEGF, and thrombocytosis

19.8 % (range: 7.0–40.6 %) from the baseline ($P < 0.001$) and leucocytosis was observed in nearly one-third of the cohort. A significant reduction in albumin (median reduction 1.9 g/dL, range: 0.5–2.7; $P < 0.001$) was also observed [22]. Eosinophilia, a hallmark of Gleich's syndrome [13] or thrombocytosis, is not typically observed. Monoclonal protein studies are indicative of an M-protein in 75–89 % of cases, and the M-protein is predominantly IgG kappa type. IgA monoclonal gammopathy associated SCLS is exceedingly uncommon [33]. The size of the M-protein is typically low. Twenty-hour urine protein electrophoresis and immunofixation studies show a monoclonal protein in nearly a third of patients. A bone marrow biopsy in patients with elevated M-protein may demonstrate a clonal plasma cell population and assist in ruling out advanced plasma cell proliferative disorders. The bone marrow plasma cell percentage is usually below 10 %, suggesting a low clonal burden as noted in MGUS. In the European registry study, eighty-nine percent of patients had evidence of concurrent monoclonal gammopathy, and in all but one patient, monoclonal gammopathy was of undetermined significance. A single case of multiple myeloma was identified [23].

Complement 1 esterase (antigen and function) assays are used to rule out hereditary angioedema [34, 35]. C3 and C4 levels can be low in nearly a quarter of the patients of SCLS. Poor renal perfusion resulting in acute renal failure can occur in up to one-half of patients, underscoring the need to closely follow the renal function during an attack [22].

Management

Acute Attacks

Owing to paucity of level 1 evidence in the management of SCLS, therapeutic strategies are dependent upon the information available through small case series or reports. The optimal management is unclear, but as the patient progresses through the distinct phases of an acute attack, specific phase-related approach is warranted. During the initial capillary leak phase, prompt institution of supportive care is imperative [22, 24]. Oral hydration with electrolyte-rich fluids should be initiated at the onset of an attack until intravenous fluids and a higher level of care are available. Admission to an intensive care unit may be required for closer monitoring of hemodynamic and metabolic parameters and management. The central venous pressure monitoring by intensivists and judicious use of vasopressors and colloids (25 % albumin, 10 % pentastarch) may avert organ dysfunction and recruitment pulmonary edema that can precipitate with overhydration. Overzealous attempts of hydration to achieve normotension should be avoided. Patients should be closely observed for the development of complications such as rhabdomyolysis, life-threatening dyselectrolytemias, compartment syndrome, deep venous thrombosis (DVT), and acute kidney injury [22, 24, 36]. Attempts to maintain adequate cerebral and renal perfusion and simultaneous prevention of fluid overload can be challenging [20].

The role of steroid therapy [18, 37, 38] during the cytokine-mediated endothelial damage is controversial [39], and steroids are best avoided in the face of a progressive flare as well as for long-term prophylaxis. Both plasmapheresis [18, 21, 40, 41] and intravenous gamma globulin (IVIG) [21, 42, 43] have been reported to successfully thwart an acute attack.

A recently proposed Severity Scale takes into account the decrease in albumin level, increase in hemoglobin, and response to therapy (Table 8.2) in patients with recurrent attacks [24]. In Grade 1 attacks, oral hydration alone is sufficient to restore normotension while grade 2 flares require outpatient management with IV fluids. Grade 3 attacks mandate hospitalization and require intensive care unit management, and Grade 4 attacks are unresponsive to therapy and uniformly fatal [24].

Prevention of Recurrent Attacks

The importance of prophylactic therapy is underscored by the data provided in the European series which displayed a five-year survival of only 20 % from diagnosis in patients not receiving any prophylactic therapy versus 85 % in the subset that received some form of prophylactic therapy [23]. A large proportion of patients (82 %) in the series received at least one of prophylactic therapies. However, the small sample size ($n = 28$) prohibited accurate ascertainment of the magnitude of benefit with this approach. With the prophylactic therapy, the median decrease in annual frequency of attack was 1.55 (range, 0.14–8.84) per patient compared to a median decrease of 0.71 attacks/patient observed in the cohort not receiving prophylactic therapy. All five patients who did not receive prophylactic therapy succumbed compared to 3/23 who received prophylactic therapy ($P < 0.001$) [23].

Beta-Adrenergic Agonists and Phosphodiesterase Inhibitors

Continuous use of beta-adrenergic agonists such as terbutaline (400 mg twice daily) and phosphodiesterase inhibitors such as theophylline (5 mg five times a day) and aminophylline [19] has the potential to increase intracellular cyclic adenosine monophosphate or inhibit intracellular Rho kinase pathway [44], reduce bradykinin- and histamine-mediated hyperpermeability, and maintain prolonged attack-free periods [20].

An initial series of 8 patients from Mayo Clinic reported efficacy of terbutaline and theophylline in reducing the severity as well as the frequency of SCLS attacks [20]. The beneficial effect was confirmed by Gousseff and Amoura in a review of 33 cases that showed an improvement in frequency of flares in nearly two-third of the patients [45]. However, nearly half of the patients who experienced an improvement in symptoms eventually relapsed. Although a therapeutic range for theophylline has not been validated in SCLS patients, prior to labeling it ineffective, and switching to another regimen, it may be useful to ensure that the levels of theophylline are in the range considered therapeutic (10–20 mg/L) in patients with asthma.

Intravenous Immunoglobulin

In the past decade, SCLS attacks have been successfully prevented or the frequency and severity of attacks reduced with the use of IVIG alone [4, 23, 43, 45–47]. Sixty-four percent of patients in the European study had received IVIG prophylactic therapy and an increase in its use has been noted in the recent years.

Table 8.2 Severity scale of an acute idiopathic systemic capillary leak syndrome attack

Severity	Hemoglobin increase and Albumin decrease	Responds to
Grade 1 A	Hgb↑ ≤ 3 g/dL Alb↓ ≤ 0.5 g/dL	Oral hydration
Grade 1 B	Hgb ↑ ≥ 3 g/dL Alb ↓ ≥ 0.5 g/dL	
Grade 2A	Hgb ↑ ≤ 3 g/dL Alb ↓ ≤ 0.5 g/dL	Outpatient intravenous fluids
Grade 2B	Hgb ↑ ≥ 3 g/dL Alb ↓ ≥ 0.5 g/dL	
Grade 3	Present, but the degree of change is not applicable	Intensive care unit monitoring
Grade 4	Present, but the degree of change is not applicable	Intractable/fatal

Adapted from Druey and Greipp [24]

MGUS-related acquired von Willebrand factor or acquired neuropathy has been shown to respond to IVIG lending further support to its use in other monoclonal gammopathy-related disorders such as SCLS. While the exact mechanism of action of IVIG in SCLS is not known, several theories including anti-idiotype effect against antibodies and blockade of Fc receptors on leukocytes, inhibition of complement-mediated damage, and prevention of SCLS triggering infections have been proposed [47, 48]. In the European study, 44 % of the patients receiving IVIG prophylactic therapy experienced no recurrent attacks after initiation of this therapy. Prophylactic IVIG is typically administered as 0.4–2 g/kg per month intravenously, and common adverse effects include infusional reactions, headaches, fatigue, and nausea. Serious side effects, including thromboembolic events, hemolytic anemia, and acute renal failure, have also been reported.

Alternative Approaches

Anecdotal reports of efficacy of verapamil [49], leukotriene inhibitors [50, 51], epoprostenol [52], immunoadsorption [50], and thalidomide [40] in SCLS have been published. Endothelial targets such as VEGF have also been exploited for therapeutic intervention. Monoclonal antibodies, bevacizumab (anti-VEGF), and infliximab (anti-TNF-α) have exhibited varying efficacy although a recent preclinical study failed to highlight any benefit of bevacizumab [2, 40, 53, 54]. Ex vivo screening for effective therapies with quantitative and humanized cell-based assays for humoral mediators of permeability has been proposed [33] as analysis of patients' cytokine profiles during attacks could potentially help tailor therapy, particularly in cases recalcitrant to commonly used agents [33].

Attacks of SCLS in patients with concomitant multiple myeloma appear to abate with the institution of anti-myeloma therapy [21], and given the dearth of highly effective anti-SCLS therapies, a case in favor of using novel anti-myeloma agent(s) even in patients with otherwise asymptomatic multiple myeloma, but coexisting SCLS, can be made.

Prognosis, Complications, and Outcome

Idiopathic SCLS has an unpredictable course. Severe attacks or complications thereof can be fatal [22, 23]. In the Mayo study, 24 % of the patients did not have recurrence of attacks for 2 years or longer. Acute renal impairment (57 % of cases) with or without rhabdomyolysis (36 %) was observed in the series. Close monitoring of creatinine, creatinine kinase, uric acid, and electrolytes is required such cases. The study indicated that greater the reduction of albumin from baseline during an attack, the higher the likelihood of developing rhabdomyolysis ($P = 0.03$). However, no such association between rhabdomyolysis and hematocrit increase was observed. Pericardial effusion (32 %), pleural effusion (28 %), seizures (8 %), and deep venous thrombosis (8 %) can also potentially result from an attack. In the European study, 75 % of patients death occurred because of SCLS related–ventricular arrhythmias, multiorgan failure, septic shock, or pericardial tamponade.

Compartment syndrome [55–58] and acute ischemic stroke are two dreaded complications with long-term sequelae. A majority of patients with compartment syndrome require fasciotomy [22, 23].

Development of cardiac tamponade may require urgent pericardiocentesis followed by pericardial window placement. Overzealous hydration in the face of normalizing capillary permeability during the recovery or recruitment phase commonly leads to an iatrogenic complication of pulmonary edema [7, 59]. In the Mayo series, recruitment pulmonary edema developed in 40 % of the patients with a few cases requiring mechanical ventilation [22].

The prognosis appears to be superior in the pediatric population [22, 60]. In the patients with abnormal monoclonal protein studies, the rate of progression to multiple myeloma appears to be no greater than that of MGUS without coexisting SCLS [22, 61]. However, lifelong surveillance for related plasma cell proliferative disorders is necessary in those with monoclonal gammopathy. Survival rate was 73–76 % at 5 years in the two major series [22, 23], reflecting an improvement in mortality when compared to previous studies [18, 21].

Summary

Diagnostic as well as therapeutic challenges encountered with the complex disorder of idiopathic SCLS can be perplexing to the patients and clinicians alike. Moreover, the attacks in SCLS are often sudden, prodromal features are non-specific, and plasma extravasation can rapidly progress, allowing little time for prompt intervention. Restoration of normal perfusion requires judicious use of vasopressors, fluids, and occasionally diuretics. Preventive therapy with beta-2 agonists, methylxanthines, or IVIG may reduce the frequency and severity of attacks. Idiopathic SCLS should invariably be excluded in all patients presenting with transient episodes of distributive shock of unclear etiology. With fewer than 200 cases reported in the literature, SCLS remains an underrecognized disorder of substantial morbidity and mortality. The need to establish greater awareness of this orphan disease among clinicians cannot be overemphasized. The treatment paradigms would continue to evolve with deeper understanding of the disease biology.

References

1. Takabatake T. Systemic capillary leak syndrome. Intern Med. 2002;41 (11):909–10.
2. Lesterhuis WJ, Rennings AJ, Leenders WP, Nooteboom A, Punt CJ, Sweep FC, et al. Vascular endothelial growth factor in systemic capillary leak syndrome. Am J Med. 2009;122(6):e5–7.
3. Xie Z, Ghosh CC, Patel R, Iwaki S, Gaskins D, Nelson C, et al. Vascular endothelial hyperpermeability induces the clinical symptoms of Clarkson disease (the systemic capillary leak syndrome). Blood. 2012;119 (18):4321–32. [Research Support, N.I.H., Extramural Research Support, N.I.H., Intramural].
4. Vigneau C, Haymann JP, Khoury N, Sraer JD, Rondeau E. An unusual evolution of the systemic capillary leak syndrome. Nephrol Dial Transplant. 2002;17(3):492–4.
5. Dhir V, Arya V, Malav IC, Suryanarayanan BS, Gupta R, Dey AB. Idiopathic systemic capillary leak syndrome (SCLS): case report and systematic review of cases reported in the last 16 years. Intern Med. 2007;46(12):899–904.
6. Bonadies N, Baud P, Peter HJ, Buergi U, Mueller BU. A case report of Clarkson's disease: If you don't know it, you'll miss it. Eur J Intern Med. 2006;17(5):363–5.
7. Chihara R, Nakamoto H, Arima H, Moriwaki K, Kanno Y, Sugahara S, et al. Systemic capillary leak syndrome. Intern Med. 2002;41(11):953–6.
8. Ghosh K, Madkaikar M, Iyer Y, Pathare A, Jijina F, Mohanty D. Systemic capillary leak syndrome preceding plasma cell leukaemia. Acta Haematol. 2001;106(3):118–21.
9. Kawabe S, Saeki T, Yamazaki H, Nagai M, Aoyagi R, Miyamura S. Systemic capillary leak syndrome. Intern Med. 2002;41(3):211–5.
10. Abdul-Ghaffar NU, Farghaly MM, Swamy AS. Acute renal failure, compartment syndrome, and systemic capillary leak syndrome complicating carbon monoxide poisoning. J Toxicol Clin Toxicol. 1996;34(6):713–9.
11. Clarkson B, Thompson D, Horwith M, Luckey EH. Cyclical edema and shock due to increased capillary permeability. Am J Med. 1960;29:193–216.
12. Preston GM, Rees JR, Spathis GS. A man with cyclical oedema. Guys Hosp Rep. 1962;111:69–79.
13. Gleich GJ, Schroeter AL, Marcoux JP, Sachs MI, O'Connell EJ, Kohler PF. Episodic angioedema associated with eosinophilia. N Engl J Med. 1984;310(25):1621–6.
14. Banerji A, Weller PF, Sheikh J. Cytokine-associated angioedema syndromes including episodic angioedema with eosinophilia (Gleich's Syndrome). Immunol Allergy Clin North Am. 2006;26(4):769–81.
15. Weinbren I. Spontaneous periodic oedema. A new syndrome. Lancet. 1963;2(7307):544–6.

16. Horwith M, Hagstrom JW, Riggins RC, Luckey EH. Hypovolemic shock and edema due to increased capillary permeability. JAMA. 1967;200 (2):101–4.

17. Atkinson JP, Waldmann TA, Stein SF, Gelfand JA, Macdonald WJ, Heck LW, et al. Systemic capillary leak syndrome and monoclonal IgG gammopathy; studies in a sixth patient and a review of the literature. Medicine (Baltimore). 1977;56(3):225–39.

18. Teelucksingh S, Padfield PL, Edwards CR. Systemic capillary leak syndrome. Q J Med. 1990;75(277):515–24.

19. Droder RM, Kyle RA, Greipp PR. Control of systemic capillary leak syndrome with aminophylline and terbutaline. Am J Med. 1992;92(5):523–6.

20. Tahirkheli NK, Greipp PR. Treatment of the systemic capillary leak syndrome with terbutaline and theophylline. A case series. Ann Intern Med. 1999;130(11):905–9.

21. Amoura Z, Papo T, Ninet J, Hatron PY, Guillaumie J, Piette AM, et al. Systemic capillary leak syndrome: report on 13 patients with special focus on course and treatment. Am J Med. 1997;103(6):514–9.

22. Kapoor P, Greipp PT, Schaefer EW, Mandrekar SJ, Kamal AH, Gonzalez-Paz NC, et al. Idiopathic systemic capillary leak syndrome (Clarkson's disease): the Mayo clinic experience. Mayo Clin Proc. 2010;85 (10):905–12. [Comparative Study].

23. Gousseff M, Arnaud L, Lambert M, Hot A, Hamidou M, Duhaut P, et al. The systemic capillary leak syndrome: a case series of 28 patients from a European registry. Ann Intern Med. 2011;154(7):464–71. [Research Support, Non-U.S. Gov't].

24. Druey KM, Greipp PR. Narrative review: the systemic capillary leak syndrome. Ann Intern Med. 2010;153(2):90–8. [Research Support, N.I.H., Extramural Research Support, N.I.H., Intramural Review].

25. Cicardi M, Gardinali M, Bisiani G, Rosti A, Allavena P, Agostoni A. The systemic capillary leak syndrome: appearance of interleukin-2-receptor-positive cells during attacks. Ann Intern Med. 1990;113(6):475–7.

26. Assaly R, Olson D, Hammersley J, Fan PS, Liu J, Shapiro JI, et al. Initial evidence of endothelial cell apoptosis as a mechanism of systemic capillary leak syndrome. Chest. 2001;120(4):1301–8.

27. Hsiao SC, Wang MC, Chang H, Pei SN. Recurrent capillary leak syndrome following bortezomib therapy in a patient with relapsed myeloma. Ann Pharmacother. 2010;44(3):587–9. [Case Reports].

28. Beermann W, Horstrup KA, Will R. Systemic capillary leak syndrome. Am J Med. 1998;105(6):554.

29. Zhang W, Ewan PW, Lachmann PJ. The paraproteins in systemic capillary leak syndrome. Clin Exp Immunol. 1993;93(3):424–9.

30. Xie Z, Nagarajan V, Sturdevant DE, Iwaki S, Chan E, Wisch L, et al. Genome-wide SNP analysis of the Systemic Capillary Leak Syndrome (Clarkson disease). Rare Dis. 2013;1(1).

31. Sion-Sarid R, Lerman-Sagie T, Blumkin L, Ben-Ami D, Cohen I, Houri S. Neurologic involvement in a child with systemic capillary leak syndrome. Pediatrics. 2010;125(3):e687–92. [Case Reports].

32. Airaghi L, Montori D, Santambrogio L, Miadonna A, Tedeschi A. Chronic systemic capillary leak syndrome. Report of a case and review of the literature. J Intern Med. 2000;247(6):731–5.
33. Xie Z, Ghosh CC, Parikh SM, Druey KM. Mechanistic classification of the systemic capillary leak syndrome: Clarkson disease. Am J Respir Crit Care Med. 2014;189(9):1145–7. [Letter Research Support, N.I.H., Extramural Research Support, N.I.H., Intramural Research Support, Non-U.S. Gov't].
34. Bracho FA. Hereditary angioedema. Curr Opin Hematol. 2005;12(6):493–8.
35. Lofdahl CG, Solvell L, Laurell AB, Johansson BR. Systemic capillary leak syndrome with monoclonal IgG and complement alterations. A case report on an episodic syndrome. Acta Med Scand. 1979;206(5):405–12.
36. Dolberg-Stolik OC, Putterman C, Rubinow A, Rivkind AI, Sprung CL. Idiopathic capillary leak syndrome complicated by massive rhabdomyolysis. Chest. 1993;104(1):123–6.
37. Kao NL, Richmond GW, Luskin AT. Systemic capillary leak syndrome. Chest. 1993;104(5):1637–8.
38. Fardet L, Kerob D, Rybojad M, Vignon-Pennamen MD, Schlemmer B, Guermazi A, et al. Idiopathic systemic capillary leak syndrome: cutaneous involvement can be misleading. Dermatology. 2004;209(4):291–5.
39. Cicardi M, Berti E, Caputo V, Radice F, Gardinali M, Agostoni A. Idiopathic capillary leak syndrome: evidence of CD8-positive lymphocytes surrounding damaged endothelial cells. J Allergy Clin Immunol. 1997;99 (3):417–9.
40. Staak JO, Glossmann JP, Esser JM, Diehl V, Mietz H, Josting A. Thalidomide for systemic capillary leak syndrome. Am J Med. 2003;115 (4):332–4.
41. Ewan PW, Lachmann PJ, Morice AH, Forster PJG. Treatment of systemic capillary leak syndrome. Lancet. 1988;332:1496.
42. Lassoued K, Clauvel JP, Similowski T, Autran B, Bengoufa D, Oksenhendler E. Pulmonary infections associated with systemic capillary leak syndrome attacks in a patient with hypogammaglobulinemia. Intensive Care Med. 1998;24(9):981–3.
43. Lambert M, Launay D, Hachulla E, Morell-Dubois S, Soland V, Queyrel V, et al. High-dose intravenous immunoglobulins dramatically reverse systemic capillary leak syndrome. Crit Care Med. 2008;36 (7):2184–7.
44. van Niew Amerongen GP, va Hinsburgh VW. Targets for pharmacological intervention of endothelial hyperpermeability and barrier function. Vascul Pharmacol. 2002;39(4–5):257–72.
45. Gousseff M, Amoura Z. [Idiopathic capillary leak syndrome]. Rev Med Interne. 2009;30(9):754–68. [Comparative Study Review].
46. Abgueguen P, Chennebault JM, Pichard E. Immunoglobulins for treatment of systemic capillary leak syndrome. The American journal of medicine. 2010;123(6):e3–4. [Case Reports Letter].
47. Zipponi M, Eugster R, Birrenbach T. High-dose intravenous immunoglobulins: a promising therapeutic approach for idiopathic systemic capillary leak syndrome. BMJ Case Rep. 2011;2011. [Case Reports].

48. Lassoued K, Clauvel JP, Similowski T, Autran B, Bengoufa D, Oksenhendler E. Pulmonary infections associated with systemic capillary leak syndrome attacks in a patient with hypogammaglobulinemia. Intensive Care Med. 1998;24(9):981–3. [Case Reports].

49. Kang PM, Lawrence C, Khan GA, Hays RM. Fulminating systemic capillary leak syndrome with lymphocytosis and hypogammaglobulinemia. Ren Fail. 1995;17(5):615–7.

50. Walinder O, Einarsson P, Lindberger K. [A case report of systemic capillary leak syndrome. Effective treatment with immunoadsorption and leukotriene antagonist] Article in Swedish. Lakartidningen. 2004;101 (38):2880–2.

51. Lilly CM, Silverman ES, Sheffer AL. Systemic capillary leak syndrome, leukotrienes, and anaphylaxis. J Intensive Care Med. 2002;17:189–94.

52. Fellows IW, Powell RJ, Toghill PJ, Williams TJ, Cohen GF. Epoprostenol in systemic capillary leak syndrome. Lancet. 1988;2(8620):1143.

53. Dowden AM, Rullo OJ, Aziz N, Fasano MB, Chatila T, Ballas ZK. Idiopathic systemic capillary leak syndrome: novel therapy for acute attacks. J Allergy Clin Immunol. 2009;124(5):1111–3.

54. Yabe H, Yabe M, Koike T, Shimizu T, Morimoto T, Kato S. Rapid improvement of life-threatening capillary leak syndrome after stem cell transplantation by bevacizumab. Blood. [Case Reports Letter]. 2010 Apr 1;115(13):2723–4.

55. Guidet B, Guerin B, Maury E, Offenstadt G, Amstutz P. Capillary leakage complicated by compartment syndrome necessitating surgery. Intensive Care Med. 1990;16(5):332–3.

56. Milner CS, Wagstaff MJ, Rose GK. Compartment syndrome of multiple limbs: An unusual presentation. J Plast Reconstr Aesthet Surg. 2006;59 (11):1251–2.

57. Prieto Valderrey F, Burillo Putze G, Martinez Azario J, Santana Ramos M. Systemic capillary leak syndrome associated with rhabdomyolysis and compartment syndrome. Am J Emerg Med. 1999;17(7):743–4.

58. Sanghavi R, Aneman A, Parr M, Dunlop L, Champion D. Systemic capillary leak syndrome associated with compartment syndrome and rhabdomyolysis. Anaesth Intensive Care. 2006;34(3):388–91.

59. Bouhaja B, Somrani N, Thabet H, Zhioua M, Yacoub M. Adult respiratory distress syndrome complicating a systemic capillary leak syndrome. Intensive Care Med. 1994;20(4):307–8.

60. Karatzios C, Gauvin F, Egerszegi EP, Tapiero B, Buteau C, Rivard GE, et al. Systemic capillary leak syndrome presenting as recurrent shock. Pediatr Crit Care Med. 2006;31:31.

61. Kyle RA, Therneau TM, Rajkumar SV, Offord JR, Larson DR, Plevak MF, et al. A long-term study of prognosis in monoclonal gammopathy of undetermined significance. N Engl J Med. 2002;346(8):564–9.

62. Estival JL, Dupin M, Kanitakis J, Combemale P. Capillary leak syndrome induced by acitretin. Br J Dermatol. 2004;150(1):150–2.

63. Rechner I, Brito-Babapulle F, Fielden J. Systemic capillary leak syndrome after granulocyte colony-stimulating factor (G-CSF). Hematol J. 2003;4 (1):54–6.

64. Talpur R, Apisarnthanarax N, Ward S, Duvic M. Treatment of refractory peripheral T-cell lymphoma with denileukin diftitox (ONTAK). Leuk Lymphoma. 2002;43(1):121–6.
65. Yamamoto K, Mizuno M, Tsuji T, Amano T. Capillary leak syndrome after interferon treatment for chronic hepatitis C. Arch Intern Med. 2002;162(4):481–2.
66. Biswas S, Nik S, Corrie PG. Severe gemcitabine-induced capillary-leak syndrome mimicking cardiac failure in a patient with advanced pancreatic cancer and high-risk cardiovascular disease. Clin Oncol (R Coll Radiol). 2004;16(8):577–9.
67. De Pas T, Curigliano G, Franceschelli L, Catania C, Spaggiari L, de Braud F. Gemcitabine-induced systemic capillary leak syndrome. Ann Oncol. 2001;12(11):1651–2.
68. Doubek M, Brychtova Y, Tomiska M, Mayer J. Idiopathic systemic capillary leak syndrome misdiagnosed and treated as polycythemia vera. Acta Haematol. 2005;113(2):150–1.
69. Dispenzieri A, Kyle RA, Lacy MQ, Rajkumar SV, Therneau TM, Larson DR, et al. POEMS syndrome: definitions and long-term outcome. Blood. 2003;101(7):2496–506.

Chapter 9
Renal Disease Associated with Monoclonal Gammopathy

Nelson Leung, MD and Samih H. Nasr, MD

Nearly 60 years after the description of the Bence-Jones protein, Alfred von Decastello described the plugging of renal tubules by an amorphous substance in a patient who died of multiple myeloma [1]. This was one of the first descriptions of a kidney disease resulting from a monoclonal protein which later became known as "cast nephropathy." Since cast nephropathy almost always occur with multiple myeloma, the term myeloma kidney became synonymously used. Indeed, one study noted that only 3 % of myeloma patients with renal impairment had low tumor burden [2]. However, this association between a malignant condition and a kidney disease is not entirely accurate. First, cast nephropathy can be seen in patients with chronic lymphocytic leukemia (CLL) or lymphoplasmacytic lymphoma with Waldenström's macroglobulinemia (WM) [3, 4]. In addition, the human kidney diseases: cast

N. Leung, MD (✉)
Departments of Nephrology and Hypertension, Hematology, Mayo Clinic,
200 First Street SW, Rochester, MN 55905, USA
e-mail: leung.nelson@mayo.edu

S.H. Nasr, MD
Department of Laboratory Medicine and Pathology, Mayo Clinic,
200 First Street SW, Hilton 10-20, Rochester, MN 55905, USA
e-mail: nasr.samih@mayo.edu

© Springer Science+Business Media New York 2017
T.M. Zimmerman and S.K. Kumar (eds.),
Biology and Management of Unusual Plasma Cell Dyscrasias,
DOI 10.1007/978-1-4419-6848-7_9

nephropathy, immunoglobulin light-chain (AL) amyloidosis, monoclonal immunoglobulin deposition disease (MIDD) and light-chain Fanconi syndrome (LCFS) can be replicated by injecting just the monoclonal protein into animals [5]. Finally, except for cast nephropathy, multiple myeloma or lymphoma is not required for the development of the above kidney diseases. The evidence overwhelmingly supports the monoclonal proteins and not the tumor as the agent directly responsible for the kidney disease. This chapter will review the clinicopathologic character-istics of these renal diseases and their association with monoclonal gammopathy of renal significance.

Monoclonal Gammopathy of Renal Significance

Kidney diseases, once linked to multiple myeloma or lymphoma, are now recognized to be capable of developing independently of the malignancy. Only about 15 % of AL amyloidosis and 20–65 % of MIDD patients meet criteria for multiple myeloma or lymphoma [6–8]. Many of these patients never progress to multiple myeloma [9]. In fact, their biology is more similar to monoclonal gam-mopathy of undetermined significance (MGUS) or smoldering multiple myeloma than multiple myeloma. However, the use of the term MGUS in these patients is problematic and confusing. First, the term MGUS denotes undetermined significance and requires the absence of end-organ damage. In these patients, the signifi-cance of kidney damage has been established. Furthermore, the current guidelines regarding the treatment of plasma cell disorders clearly recommend against treating patients with MGUS [10]. This makes sense in true MGUS patients where there is no end-organ damage and the transformation rate to multiple myeloma or other more serious conditions is low. This is not applicable to patients who have pathologic lesions attributable to their monoclonal gammopathy. The conflicts created by the term MGUS make it inappropriate for these patients. As a result, a new term monoclonal gammopathy of renal significance (MGRS) has been created to better classify these patients and avoid confusion.

The main difference between MGRS and MGUS is the presence of a kidney disease that is attributable to the monoclonal protein [11]. Both conditions are characterized by less than 10 % clonal plasma cells in the bone marrow, <3 g/dl of monoclonal (M) protein and the absence of other defining features of multiple myeloma such as hypercalcemia, anemia, and bone lesions. However, where there is no end-organ damage in MGUS, the kidney is injured by the monoclonal protein in MGRS. This is most often as a result of deposition of monoclonal immunoglobins, but monoclonal protein can also injure the kidney by other means such as activation of the complement system. Regardless of the pathophysiology, this direct link between the kidney and the monoclonal protein is what defines MGRS. By definition, cast nephropathy is not a MGRS-related kidney disease because it is almost always associated with multiple myeloma [2, 12].

MGRS-Related Kidney Diseases with Organized Monoclonal Immunoglobulin Deposits

AL Amyloidosis

AL amyloidosis is a fatal systemic disease characterized by the extracellular deposition of congophilic fibrils in soft tissues [13]. The amyloid in AL is composed of monoclonal immunoglobin light chains (LC) while monoclonal immunoglobulin heavy-chain amyloid is called AH and those containing the intact components of immunoglobulin light and heavy chain are ALH [14, 15]. AL is by far the most common subtype representing over 95 % of the cases of immunoglobulin amyloidosis and for the purpose of this chapter will represent all of the subtypes of immunoglobulin amyloidosis. The pathogenesis is the result of the misfolding of immunoglobulin LCs into a lower energy state. The misfolded LC self-aggregates to form fibrils, which are more resistant to degradation. These are deposited in various organs. There is increasing evidence to suggest that cellular toxicity cannot be entirely explained by deposition. In a zebra fish model, impaired cardiac function, pericardial edema, and increased cell death can be induced by the introduction of amy-loidogenic LC but not control LC from myeloma patients [16]. These changes are observed prior to any fibril formation. In addition, divergent phenotypic changes are observed in mesangial cells incubated with LC from patients with AL amyloidosis versus LC from MIDD patients [17]. This data strongly suggest the toxicity is determined by the primary sequence of the LC. Finally, repeat renal biopsy of patients treated with autologous stem cell transplantation shows no regression of the amyloid deposits despite achievement of a complete hematologic response (CR) and significant improvement in proteinuria [18].

AL amyloidosis is the most common glomerular lesion in patients with MM [19, 20]. It is found in 5–15 % of patients with MM at autopsy [19, 21, 22]. However, only a small percentage of patients actually have multiple myeloma. In a study of 474 patients, 22 % of patients have 10–19 % plasma cells while 18 % of patients have >20 % plasma cells in the bone marrow [6]. Seven percent of patients have >3 g/dl of M protein in the serum. Only 9.5 % met criteria for MM, and they all had lytic bone lesions. Median age of patients with AL amyloidosis is 64 years, and 69 % are male. The light chains are not equally represented as 70 % of the M-proteins are lambda restricted. AL amyloidosis has also been reported to occur in B-cell lymphoproliferative disorders and CLL [23, 24].

In systemic AL amyloidosis, kidney is the most commonly involved organ. An abnormal creatinine is seen in nearly half of the patients. Proteinuria and nephrotic syndrome are noted in 73 and 28 %, respectively [6]. Median proteinuria is 5.8 g/d. The pro-teinuria is mainly albuminuria, which makes up on average 70 % of the urinary proteins [25]. In a small percentage of patients, a vascular-limited AL amyloidosis has been described, which presents with progressive renal insufficiency but little (<1 g/d) or no proteinuria [26]. Rare patients may present with nephrogenic diabetes insipidus [6]. End-stage renal disease (ESRD) mainly developed in those who presented with renal manifestations. In a study of 145 patients, ESRD developed in 41.6 % of patients who presented with renal manifestations versus 4.9 % without [27]. ESRD appeared to negative impact survival as the median survival was 10.4 months after the start of dialysis.

The diagnosis of AL amyloidosis requires a biopsy. In the kidney, amyloid appears as an amorphous periodic acid–Schiff (PAS)-negative and silver-negative deposits (Fig. 9.1). By definition, amyloid deposits regardless of type are Congo red positive and exhibit an apple green birefringence when viewed under polarized light. Amyloid deposits are seen in glomeruli and vessels in the vast majority of cases and in the interstitium in more than half of cases. Glomerular involvement leads to mesangial expansion, which may show nodular appearance at times. When amyloid affects the glomerular basement membrane, it usually forms spicules, a characteristic feature of this disease, which can be readily identified on silver stain. For AL, the deposits should stain for a single LC by immunofluorescence (IF) (Fig. 9.1). A single heavy chain would also stain positive in ALH while only the heavy chain will stain in AH. Amyloid fibrils have a diameter of 7–12 nm and are randomly arranged when viewed by electron microscopy (EM) (Fig. 9.1). Since only amyloidosis of immunoglobulin subtypes are treated with chemotherapy, typing of the amyloid is essential prior to initiation of treatment [28]. While IF can be quite informative for AL and its subtypes, laser microdissection followed by proteomics by mass spectrometry (LM-MS) has become the gold standard and should be performed in equivocal or uncertain cases [14].

Tremendous advances have been made in the treatment of AL amyloidosis in the past decades. During this time, overall survival has increased from 18 months to over 5 years [29–32]. Details regarding treatment are covered in other chapters. What is important to note is that response in the kidney is associated with patient survival. Using a 50 % reduction in proteinuria as a marker of response, renal response was strongly associated with patient survival [33]. In subgroup analysis, patients who achieved 75 % or more proteinuria reduction were the ones who benefitted in overall survival and those who achieved 95 % reduction had the best outcomes [34]. Patients who had between 50 and 74 % reduction in proteinuria did not show an improvement in OS as compared to those who had <50 % reduction in proteinuria. Of note, the reduction in proteinuria can take 10–12 months to occur [35]. More rapid method of assessment of renal response is currently being investigated.

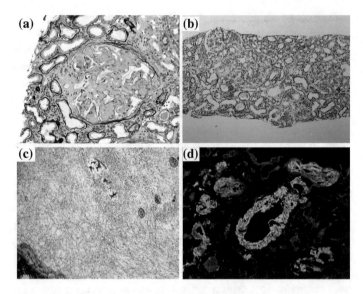

Fig. 9.1 Pathology of renal AL amyloidosis. **a** There is extensive, global mesangial, and segmental glomerular capillary wall deposition of acellular, silver-negative amyloid deposits (jones methenamine silver, ×400). **b** The figure shows global glomerular Congo red-positive amyloid, which exhibits *red/yellow/green* colors when viewed under polarized light (×100). **c** On electron microscopy, amyloid fibrils appear haphazardly oriented and measure between 7 and 12 nm in diameter (×46,000). **d** On immunofluorescence, amyloid deposits appear smudgy and stain for one of the light chains only. The figure shows smudgy transmural, arterial, and arteriolar staining for lambda (×200). Staining for kappa was negative (not shown)

Immunotactoid Glomerulonephritis

Immunotactoid glomerulonephritis (ITG) is a rare kidney disease characterized by the deposition of microtubules in the glomerulus [36]. Unlike amyloid, these fibrils are much larger and do not stain with Congo red. The average diameter of immunotactoid fibrils is 38.2 nm with a range of 20–55 nm (Fig. 9.2). The most distinguishing feature, however, is the hollow center, which is similar to microtubules. Other fibrils with similar features are cryoglobulins, thus by definition, cryoglobulinemia must be ruled out. Historically, fibrillary glomerulonephritis has been described together with ITG and was once thought to the same disease.

Histologically, they do share common features such as membranoproliferative pattern (Fig. 9.2) with endocapillary proliferation, mesangial expansion and hypercellularity, membranous-like pattern (Fig. 9.2), even hyaline pseudothrombi in the glomeruli and crescents [20, 37, 38]. Major differences include smaller fibril size in fibrillary glomerulonephritis. The fibrils are solid and randomly arranged in fibrillary glomerulonephritis whereas the microtubules in ITG are hollow and usually arranged in parallel arrays (Fig. 9.2) [37]. More importantly, ITG microtubules are commonly composed of entire monoclonal immunoglobulins while fibrillary glomerulonephritis is rarely monoclonal [39].

Clinically, patients with ITG present with heavy proteinuria. Median proteinuria is 11.1 g/d with a range of 1.4–36 g/d [20, 37, 38]. Microscopic hematuria is often present. Renal impairment is often mild with a median serum creatinine (SCr) at presentation of 1.5 mg/dl (0.7–3.8 mg/dl). The percentage of male patients ranges from 71.4 to 83.0 %, and the median age is from 59 to 66 years. Monoclonal gammopathy is present in 63–86 % of cases. One unique characteristic of ITG is the high rate of CLL reported in these patients. It can be up to 50 % in some series. Multiple myeloma was found in 12.5 % of cases in another series [40]. There are currently no clinical trials on ITG. Cytotoxic agents capable of reducing the clone have been found to be successful at preserving renal function [37].

Light-Chain Fanconi Syndrome

Light-chain Fanconi syndrome (LCFS) is a rare condition characterized by electrolyte abnormalities as a result of proximal tubular injury. The tubular injury is due to intracellular crystalline deposition of monoclonal light chains. Fanconi syndrome and proximal tubular cytoplasmic crystals may also be present in crystal-storing histiocytosis (CSH). The latter, however, is different from LCFS in that the crystals are mainly seen within the cytoplasm of histiocytes in the renal interstitium, bone marrow, and other organs. Like CSH, nearly 90 % of the cases of LCFS are kappa restricted with V_{kI} being the most common subtype [41, 42]. Multiple myeloma is

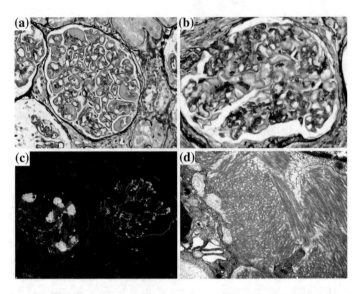

Fig. 9.2 Pathology of immunotactoid glomerulonephritis. **a** In this case of immunotactoid glomerulonephritis and a membranoproliferative pattern of injury, there is global mesangial and glomerular capillary wall deposition of silver-negative immune material together with widespread duplication of the glomerular basement membrane (jones methenamine silver, ×400). **b** In this case of immunotactoid glomerulonephritis with a membranous pattern of injury, the glomerular basement membrane appears thickened and shows global silver-positive spikes (jones methenamine silver, ×400). **c** In this case of immunotactoid glomerulonephritis, there is bright glomerular capillary wall, mesangial, and intraluminal staining for IgG (immunofluorescence, ×200). Similar glomerular staining for lambda is seen, with negative staining for kappa (not shown). **d** Electron microscopy from a case of immunotactoid glomerulopathy shows mesangial deposits composed of large microtubules with hollow centers, which are organized in parallel arrays. The microtubules measured 52 nm in mean thickness (×24,500)

diagnosed in about half of the patients with smaller percentage of patients diagnosed with WM, CLL, smoldering MM, and MGRS.

LCFS patients often present in their sixth decade with a median age of 57 years. It is slightly more common in men with 58 % male. Typical presentation includes tubular proteinuria (usually not high grade), glycosuria, and renal insufficiency. Extrarenal manifestations include bone pain, osteomalacia, and fatigue. Insufficiency fractures are not uncommon. Many patients will also have electrolyte abnormalities such as hypouricemia (66 %), hypophosphatemia (50 %), and hypokalemia (44 %), but these tend to disappear as the renal function declines [41]. One clue may be normal levels of uric acid, potassium, and phosphorus despite advanced degree of chronic kidney disease. Diagnostically, aminoaciduria (100 %) is the most common urinary abnormality followed by glycosuria (~ 100 %) and phosphaturia (43 %). Patients who have aminoaciduria but no glycosuria or phosphaturia are considered to have an incomplete Fanconi syndrome.

On kidney biopsy, elongated hypereosinophilic and PAS-negative crystals can be identified within proximal tubular cells (Fig. 9.3), usually accompanied by patchy tubular injury and varying degrees of tubular atrophy and interstitial fibrosis. Occasionally, proximal tubular cells appear swollen by the crystals [42]. Toluidine blue is the best stain for the identification of crystals. Only a single immunoglobulin LC should be present on IF (Fig. 9.3). On EM, rhomboid or rod-shaped crystals are seen in the cytoplasm (Fig. 9.3). Cast nephropathy is not uncommonly seen coexisting within the same biopsy.

The renal outcome in LCFS is variable. The percentage of patients reaching ESRD ranged from 15.6 to 72.7 % [41, 42]. It was interesting that one study found the presence of multiple myeloma was not a risk factor for ESRD [41]. Unfortunately, interpretation of the data regarding treatment had been difficult. Since most of the data came from the melphalan and prednisone era, patients who underwent treatment often did worse due to infection and other complications. Furthermore, treatment did not seem to improve renal function. The results may be quite different with the use of novel agents. There are reports of 2 patients improving after treatment with bortezomib-based therapy [43]. Both had a significant reduction in their serum kappa FLC levels.

The term light-chain proximal tubulopathy should be discussed, and it is often associated with LCFS in the literature but the precise definition has yet to be unified. Sometimes, it refer to LCFS without crystals while in others, it is used to describe light-chain crystal deposition but the absence or presence of just a partial Fanconi syndrome [44, 45]. Some feel LCFS and light-chain proximal tubulopathy are the same entity while others feel they are separate [46, 47]. One series found that light-chain proximal tubulopathy without crystals represented 3.2 % of cases of light-chain-related renal diseases, compared to 0.9 % for light-chain proximal tubulopathy with crystals [45]. In this series, 9 of the 10 cases with light-chain proximal tubulopathy without crystals were composed of lambda light chain that is opposite of what one would expect for LCFS. Patients exhibited lysosomal abnormalities (some of which had a mottled appearance) along with signs of acute tubular injury such as cytoplasmic swelling, blebbing or flattening with dilatation of tubular lumen and loss of brush border. Multiple myeloma was diagnosed in 8 of 13 patients who were diagnosed with light chain proximal tubulopathy. In another series of 190 biopsies of patients with multiple myeloma, only 1 was diagnosed as light-chain proximal tubulopathy with crystals [20]. Clearly, more research is needed in order to better define the entity of light-chain proximal tubulopathy.

Cryoglobulinemia

Cryoglobulins have the characteristic of reversibly precipitating in cold temperatures. They are composed of immunoglobulins. Three types of cryoglobulins have been identified. In type I, the immunoglobulin is monoclonal, often IgM but it can also be IgG or IgA [48]. Type II involves a monoclonal immunoglobulin most commonly IgM with affinity toward polyclonal immunoglobulins. This is often referred to as rheumatoid factor activity. Type III is composed of polyclonal immunoglobulin. Only types I and II can be considered to be MGRS and only if they are not the result of a lymphoma or multiple myeloma. Type I is the result of a B-cell lymphoproliferative disorders. Most commonly, it occurs in lymphoplasmacytic lymphoma with WM, but can be seen in multiple myeloma and CLL [48]. The most common causes of type II cryoglobulinemia are infections and autoimmune diseases but a lymphoproliferative disorder producing a monoclonal IgM will also result in type II cryoglobulinemia. The number one infectious cause of type II cryoglobulinemia in the world is hepatitis C infection, accounting for as many as 73 % of cases in some series [49].

Clinical manifestations are the result of precipitation, hyperviscosity, and leukoclastic vasculitis due to the cryoglobulins [48]. Manifestations can range from cutaneous rash and ulcers, to

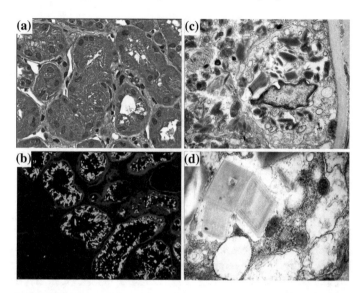

Fig. 9.3 Pathology of light-chain proximal tubulopathy. **a** Large rhomboid and rod-shaped hypereosinophilic crystals are seen within proximal tubular cells. (H&E, ×600). **b** Proximal tubular cell crystals stain strongly for kappa by immunofluorescence performed on pronase-digested, paraffin-embedded tissue (×400). The crystals were negative for lambda. C&D are from a different case of light-chain proximal tubulopathy. The proximal tubular cells are loaded with electron-dense non-membrane-bound light-chain crystals with rhomboid, rod or rectangular shapes (electron microscopy, ×13,500 for **c** and 33,000 for **d**)

neuropathy, arthritis, acrocyanosis, and Raynaud's to acral ischemia. In the kidney, cryoglobulinemia presents as glomerulonephritis with or without endovasculitis. The most common histologic pattern is membranoproliferative glomerulonephritis, but mesangioproliferative and endocapillary proliferative glomerulonephritis are also frequently observed (Fig. 9.4). Even membranous pattern has been reported. Florid monocytic infiltration of glomeruli is typical of cryoglobulinemic glomerulonephritis. Cryoglobulins can be seen forming pseudothrombi in the lumen of glomerular capillaries (Fig. 9.4) and may also be seen in the intima and lumina of arterioles and interlobular arteries, occasionally causing endovasculitis. On IF, the deposits should stain for the monoclonal immunoglobulin involved in the cryoglobulin (Fig. 9.4). C3 can also be detected. Most patients present with proteinuria and moderate renal insufficiency [49]. Only 20 % of patients have nephrotic syndrome at presentation. Another 20–30 % may present with a nephritic picture with macro- or micro-hematuria. A small percentage will present like a rapidly progressive glomerulonephritis (RPGN) with quick loss of renal function. One striking feature of cryoglobulinemia is severe hypertension. Hypertension associated with cryoglobulinemia is often difficult control. In fact, studies have found only 15 % of patients with cryoglobulinemia died of renal failure, but they are much more likely to die of cardiovascular complications or infection [49].

Treatment of cryoglobulinemia depends on the type and etiology. Anti-viral therapy has been effective for type II cryoglobulinemia secondary to hepatis C [49]. This can be combined with rituximab in severe cases [50]. Rituximab can also be used in type II secondary to autoimmune diseases and type I secondary to a lymphoproliferative disorder [49]. Plasmapheresis can be an effective adjuvant therapy to reduce hyperviscosity and ischemia. A known complication of rituximab is cryoglobulin flare. While most cases are benign and it does not denote treatment failure, the flare can result in typical complications of cryoglobulinemia [51]. Plasmapheresis and additional immunosuppressive therapy may be needed to treat the flare.

MGRS-Related Kidney Diseases with Non-organized Monoclonal Immunoglobulin Deposits

Monoclonal Immunoglobulin Deposition Disease

MIDD represents a group of kidney diseases characterized by deposits of monoclonal immunoglobulin and its components. They include light-chain deposition disease (LCDD), light- and heavy-chain deposition disease (LHCDD), and heavy-chain deposition disease (HCDD) [7]. LCDD is the most common subtype of MIDD. MIDD is seen in 5 % of MM patients in autopsy series at approximately half the incidence of AL amyloidosis [19]. The kidney is almost universally affected while systemic involvement in the lungs, heart, liver, and other soft tissue is less common and often asymptomatic [52]. The most common malignant condition associated with MIDD is multiple myeloma occurring in 59–65 % of cases while CLL is found in 3 % [7, 8]. In the past, the remainder of patients was described as idiopathic [8]. However, a recent study found 100 % of the patients with MIDD had an abnormal serum FLC ratio suggesting that these patients would be more accurately classified as MGRS [7, 11].

The most characteristic histological lesion in MIDD is nodular mesangial sclerosis [7, 53–55]. On light microscopy, these nodules are PAS and silver positive similar to Kimmelstiel–Wilson nodules of diabetic nephropathy (Fig. 9.5). Other features include mesangial sclerosis without nodules, membranoproliferative pattern, and crescents. The deposits in MIDD are Congo red negative. The most distinguishing features are seen on IF where monoclonal light chains, heavy chains or entire immunoglobulin can be seen in a linear pattern along the GBM and even more consistently along the tubular basement membranes (TBM) (Fig. 9.5). Staining of the immunoglobulin components can be seen in the mesangium, but it is less consistent than the TBM or GBM. C3 may also be detected in cases of LCHDD and HCDD. The deposits should not have any organized structure on EM and should appear as powdery or amorphous electron-dense deposits in the same compartment as seen on IF (Fig. 9.5). Occasionally, small fibers have been described.

Kappa is more commonly represented in LCDD. In opposite proportion to AL amyloidosis, 75 % of MIDD cases are due to a kappa clones [7, 8, 55, 56]. Even within the kappa light-chain family, the V_{kI} subtype seems to be most common [57]. A potential explanation may be found in its tertiary and quaternary structure. Analyses show a β-edge that is formed in the CDR2 loop of kappa light chains as a result of a conserved cis-proline at position 8 [58]. In lambda light chains, this proline is in the trans-position and it is often followed by another trans-proline at position 9 making formation the β-edge extremely unlikely. As a result of exposure of the β-edge, spontaneous aggregation of kappa light chains into oligomers has been demonstrated. These oligomers can then elongate into a fibril. These fibrils do not bind serum amyloid P

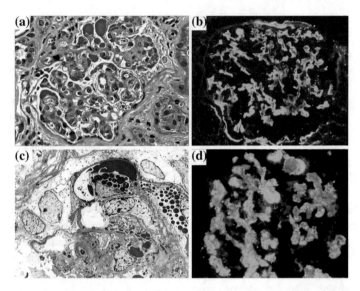

Fig. 9.4 Pathology of cryoglobulinemic glomerulonephritis. **a–d** are images from a 57-year-old female who was referred for new onset hypertension, proteinuria, and hematuria. Serum, urine, and cryoprecipitate immunofixation showed an IgG kappa monoclonal protein. Bone marrow biopsy showed 5 % plasmacytosis. **a** On light microscopy, glomeruli show mesangial hypercellularity and large glassy intracapillary hyaline thrombi "pseudothrombi," which stain bright red on trichrome stain (×400). **b** Ultrastructural examination shows large highly electron-dense subendothelial and mesangial deposits. Adjacent macrophages contain numerous phagolysosomes with the same electron density as the subendothelial deposits, consistent with phagocytosed immune material (×2000). The glomerular deposits stain brightly for IgG (**c**, ×400) and kappa (**d**, ×600) with negative lambda, trace IgM, and negative IgA (not shown) consistent with type 1 cryoglobulinemic glomerulonephritis

(SAP) or Congo red and possess no amyloid properties. It is postulated that these oligomers form the deposits that are seen in MIDD.

Median age of presentation ranged from 51 to 57 years, and roughly two-thirds of the patients were male [7, 8, 59, 60]. Proteinuria was nearly universally present with a median proteinuria of 2.7–4.1 g/d [7, 8]. Approximately 40 % of patients had nephrotic range proteinuria. Patients with HCDD present with have higher degree of proteinuria [7]. Microscopic hematuria was common (62 %), but gross hematuria was rare (3 %). Renal insufficiency was also nearly universal with an average serum creatinine of 3.8 mg/dl [7, 8]. End-stage renal disease (ESRD) was reached by 39–57 % of patients.

The prognosis of these patients is variable. One study noted a 13-month overall survival in patients with LHCDD while another showed a 90-month overall survival [7, 60]. Independent factors that influenced overall survival were age, serum creatinine at diagnosis, the presence of multiple myeloma, and the presence of lytic bone lesions [7, 8, 60]. In patients who have multiple myeloma or CLL, treatment should be specified by the disease type. Patients with MGRS should also be treated to prevent the development of ESRD. In one study, although the patient survival was 71 % at 5 years, the renal survival was only 40 %. Inadequate treatment was one of the factors leading to the high rate of ESRD. It is important to recognize that these patients do not have a malignant condition so minimizing chemotherapy-related toxicity is as important as efficacy since these patients may live for a long time with their adverse effects. Bortezomib has been shown to be effective in these patients especially with its ability to inhibit NFκB [61, 62]. The least toxic schedule and route should be employed as toxicities have been reported [63]. Autologous stem cell transplantation either alone or after induction has also produced good results [62, 64–67]. In the past, kidney transplantation in MIDD was avoided due to the high rates of recurrence ($\sim$80 %) [68]. However, patients who had achieved a hematologic complete response (CR) prior to kidney transplantation may have lower risk of recurrence and better kidney allograft outcome [65].

Membranoproliferative Glomerulonephritis with Monoclonal Deposits

Membranoproliferative glomerulonephritis (MPGN) is a group of kidney diseases that share a common histopathologic pattern of injury. MPGN traditionally had been classified by the location of the deposits. Of the three types, type II MPGN, also known as dense deposit disease (DDD), had a unique pathophysiology [69, 70]. DDD is the result of abnormal complement activation resulting in the deposition of C3 [71]. MPGN secondary to infection,

autoimmune diseases, malignancy and other complement dysregulation can present as either type I or III. The contribution of
monoclonal gammopathy in the pathogenesis of MPGN was not
recognized until recently. In a single-center study that excluded
patients with hepatitis (B & C) and DDD found 41 % of the
MPGN cases had a circulating monoclonal protein [72].
Monoclonal protein deposits were found in the kidney in most of
these patients. While majority of the cases were MGRS, 21 % met
criteria for multiple myeloma and another 17.8 % had WM, CLL,
and other lymphomas.

Histologically, MPGN is characterized by mesangial hypercellularity, endocapillary proliferation, and capillary wall remodeling
[70]. The glomeruli often appear lobular, and double contours can
be seen along the basement membranes on light microscopy.
Electron-dense immune deposits can be seen in the mesangium and
subendothelial space with or without subepithelial deposits.
Granular deposits can be seen on IF that should stain for single
heavy chain and a single light chain [72]. C3 deposits are usually
found along the capillary walls.

Renal impairment and proteinuria were the most common presentation. Median SCr was 2.5 mg/dl, and proteinuria was 3.8 g/d
[72]. Many of the patients also had microscopic hematuria.
Hypertension, which was usually mild, was common among these
patients. Complement levels were normal. Median age at presentation was 59 years with 57 % males. Limited follow-up did not
allow for long-term prognosis assessment. However, patients with
concomitant multiple myeloma appear to have the worse renal
outcomes.

Proliferative Glomerulonephritis with Monoclonal IgG Deposits

A relatively new kidney disease associated with MGRS is the
proliferative glomerulonephritis with monoclonal IgG deposits
(PGNMID) [15, 73]. A unique feature of these patients is their
preference for monoclonal IgG3. IgG3-κ accounts for more than
50 % of cases, and IgG3-λ contributes to another ~13 % of cases.
Hematologically, they tend to have a low clonal disease burden.

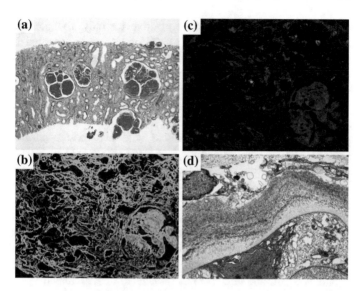

Fig. 9.5 Pathology of renal monoclonal immunoglobulin deposition disease. **a** Glomeruli have a nodular appearance due to mesangial sclerosis and massive deposition of lambda light chain. The nodules are paucicellular, glassy, and stain PAS positive, mimicking diabetic glomerulosclerosis (PAS, ×100). **b** and **c** are from the same biopsy as **a**. Immunofluorescence shows diffuse linear glomerular and tubular basement membranes and smudgy mesangial staining for lambda (**b**, ×200) with negative staining for kappa (**c**, ×200). The diagnostic ultrastructural finding in MIDD is punctate, powdery electron-dense deposits involving the inner aspect of the glomerular basement membranes (not shown) and the outer aspect of the tubular basement membranes (**d**, electron microscopy, ×9700)

Less than 10 % of patients qualify for multiple myeloma and over half do not even have detectable circulating monoclonal protein. Despite that, they have a high rate of recurrence after kidney transplantation, which has been detected as early as 3 months post-transplant [74].

On biopsy, the dominate feature is mixture of proliferative and membranoproliferative glomerulonephritis (Fig. 9.6). This is often diffuse endocapillary proliferation and leukocyte infiltration. PGNMID may show membranous features and crescents [15]. Interstitial fibrosis can be seen in more advanced cases. Glomerular capillary walls and the mesangial deposits are granular in appearance on IF and should be positive for only a single IgG subtype and light chain (Fig. 9.6). C3 and C1q are detected in glomeruli in most cases. By EM, the deposits are predominantly granular (i.e., without substructure) and are predominately subendothelial and mesangial in location (Fig. 9.6). A minority of deposits may show lattice-like array with a periodicity of 15 nm. An IgA variant has been described [75].

These patients commonly present with nephrotic syndrome (>50 %) [73]. Mean proteinuria is 5.7 g/d. Most will also have renal impairment with the median SCr of 2.8 mg/dl. Microscopic hematuria may be detected in majority of the patients. Mean age of presentation was 54 years with 62 % females. During a mean follow-up of 30 months in one study, 21.9 % of the patients developed ESRD and 15.6 % had died [73]. Response has been reported with alkylator and steroids, rituximab, and steroids alone. Experience with anti-myeloma therapy especially with novel agents is small, and effectiveness remains to be determined.

MGRS-Related Kidney Disease Without Monoclonal Immunoglobulin Deposits

C3 Glomerulonephritis

C3 glomerulonephritis (C3GN) is a subset of C3 glomerulopathy that includes DDD and CFHR3 nephropathy [76]. It is characterized by deposits that are predominate C3 and without C1q, C4 or immunoglobulins (Fig. 9.7) [77]. By light microscopy, it may show features of MPGN, mesangial proliferative glomerulonephritis or endocapillary proliferative glomerulonephritis (Fig. 9.7) It may also exhibit prominent glomerular neutrophil infiltration mimicking postinfectious glomerulonephritis. Deposits can be both subendothelial, subepithelial, and/or mesangial on EM (Fig. 9.7). The appearance is, however, less electron dense than those of immunoglobulin deposits (Fig. 9.7).

Majority of the cases of C3GN is due to dysfunctional regulation of the alternative complement pathway. This is similar to the pathophysiology of DDD [77]. However, some patients with C3GN also have circulating monoclonal protein [78, 79]. In one

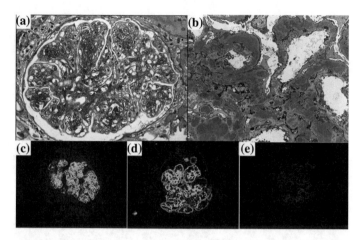

Fig. 9.6 Pathology of proliferative glomerulonephritis with monoclonal IgG deposits. **a** The glomerulus exhibits a membranoproliferative glomerulonephritis pattern of injury with moderate global mesangial hypercellularity and sclerosis, together with segmental duplication of the glomerular basement membrane and endocapillary hypercellularity (PAS, ×400). **b** On electron microscopy, there are large mesangial, intramembranous, and subendothelial deposits, together with segmental duplication of the glomerular basement membrane. The electron-dense deposits appear granular (without substructure) (×3000). **c–e** Glomeruli in this patient with PGNMID exhibit bright global mesangial and glomerular capillary wall staining for IgG3 (**c**) and kappa (**d**). Glomeruli are negative for lambda (**e**), IgA, IgM, IgG1, IgG2, and IgG4 (not shown). No extraglomerular staining for IgG or kappa is seen (×400 for **c–e**)

series, the incidence was up to 31 %. It has been shown that autoantibodies known as C3 nephritis factor (C3nef) can bind C3 convertase to stabilize it against the degradation effects of factor H [76]. These autoantibodies were typically thought to be polyclonal [80]. However, a study of 17 serum samples of patients with C3nef activity showed differential C3nef activity in samples treated with either anti-κ or anti-λ Sepharose, suggesting the possibility of monoclonal proteins acting as C3nef [81]. Indeed, monoclonal IgG and IgM C3nef have been isolated from patients with MPGN [82]. These evidences support the possibility that a monoclonal gammopathy could have C3nef activity resulting in C3GN or DDD [83].

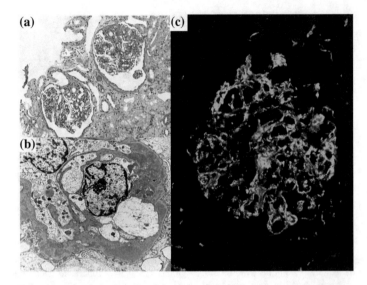

Fig. 9.7 Pathology of C3 glomerulonephritis. **a** On light microscopy, glomeruli show marked global mesangial hypercellularity (PAS, ×200). **b** On electron microscopy, there are large moderately electron-dense, ill-defined mesangial, intramembranous, and subendothelial deposits (×10,000). **c** On immunofluorescence, there is global granular mesangial and glomerular capillary wall staining for C3 (×400). Glomeruli are negative for IgG, IgA, IgM, kappa, and lambda in this case (not shown)

Thrombotic Microangiopathy in POEMS Syndrome

POEMS syndrome also known as Crow–Fukase syndrome is multisystemic disease most commonly due to a lambda-restricted monoclonal gammopathy [84]. The name POEMS is taken from 5 of the more common presentations, which include polyneuropathy, organomegaly, endocrinopathy, monoclonal gammopathy, skin manifestations, and sclerotic bone lesions [85]. Other features include extravascular volume overload, thrombocytosis, elevated levels of vascular endothelial growth factor (VEGF), and interleukin (IL)-6. The monoclonal protein is almost always lambda. This disease mimics MGUS as the median percentage of plasma cells in the bone marrow is 5 %. POEMS syndrome can also arise from smoldering multiple myeloma, plasmacytoma, lymphoplasmacytic lymphoma, and Castleman disease.

Renal manifestations are not prominent features in POEMS. Often, patients may have renal insufficiency due to issues with volume. One unique feature is asymmetric size of the kidneys, which is thought to be due to unilateral renomegaly while other feels it is due to unilateral atrophy [86]. Rare patients can develop ESRD. Renal pathology in these patients often shows an MPGN-like lesion [87]. Immunoglobulin deposits are often not found [88]. In addition to the typical mesangial and endocapillary proliferation, mesangiolysis, microaneurysm, and swelling of the endothelial cells resembling thrombotic microangiopathy are common found, but thrombi associated with microangiopathic hemolytic anemia have not been reported [87–90]. Alterations in VEGF, platelet-derived growth factor (PDGF) and IL-6 levels have been suggested as the pathogenesis but elevated levels are not consistently found in patients with renal involvement [91]. Renal response to treatment has been reported but relapses are common although no data on renal response with novel agents had been reported [87].

Recurrent Diseases After Kidney Transplantation

One common feature shared by all MGRS-related kidney disease is the high frequency of recurrence after kidney transplantation. All glomerular diseases can recur after kidney transplantation. Diseases such as membranous nephropathy and focal segmental glomerulosclerosis have recurrence rates between 7 and 50 % [92]. Recurrence of IgA nephropathy can be as high as 61 % but loss of kidney allograft is uncommon. Recurrence of ANCA-associated vasculitis is less than 10 % likely the result of immunosuppression [93]. On the other hand, MGRS-related kidney diseases can recur at >80 %. Often, this is associated with allograft loss and death of the patient, making kidney transplantation difficult.

The best example of the high recurrence rate in MGRS-related kidney diseases is MIDD. In a single-center study, 5 of 7 patients with LCDD developed recurrent disease in their renal allograft

[68]. Median time to recurrence is 33 months with a range of 3–45. Recurrence disease was associated with loss of kidney allograft and/or death. Similar experience was noted in a review of 7 patients where 6 eventually developed recurrent disease [94]. Similar results are found in patients with fibrillary glomerulonephritis. In a study of 12 patients with fibrillary glomerulonephritis, 4 of 7 patients with a monoclonal gammopathy had recurrent disease after kidney transplantation [95]. One patient had recurrence in the second allograft after losing the first allograft to recurrent disease. In comparison, patients with fibrillary glomerulonephritis but without monoclonal proteins had no recurrence. In a study of recurrent MPGN, the only factor that was predictive of recurrence was abnormal complement levels at the time of kidney transplantation [96]. However, the presence of a monoclonal gammopathy showed a trend toward significance with nearly 3 times as many recurrences in those with a monoclonal protein. No large studies have been reported for PGNMID but recurrences have been reported. Recurrence tends to be rapid in these patients with a median time to recurrence at 3.8 months [74]. Graft lost is not uncommon.

Diagnosis of MGRS-Related Kidney Diseases

The definition of MGRS requires that the monoclonal gammopathy has a direct role in the pathogenesis of the kidney disease [11]. This can only be demonstrated by a kidney biopsy. This is especially important in patients over the age of 60 where the rate of MGUS far exceeds the rate of kidney disease [97, 98]. In separate studies from the same county, the prevalence of glomerular disease was found to be 9.0/100,000 person-year while the incidence of finding a monoclonal gammopathy in persons between the ages of 60–70 was 3 and 4.6 % for those 70–80 years of age. The presence of a monoclonal gammopathy and renal insufficiency is not sufficient to make the diagnosis. The most direct way to establishing the association between the kidney disease and the monoclonal protein is to demonstrate deposition of the monoclonal protein in the kidney. This can be assessed by immunofluorescence [14]. Restriction to a single light chain and/or heavy chain is required for demonstration of monoclonality. In some cases, immunohisto-chemistry may be inconclusive. In such circumstances, proteomics by mass spectrometry has been extremely useful. In fact, mass spectrometry has become the gold standard for protein identification and typing for amyloid deposits [99]. Proving the connection between C3 deposits and a monoclonal gammopathy is more difficult. Ideally, a C3 (or C4) nephritic factor should be detected and should be identified as the monoclonal protein. This would insure that the monoclonal protein is activating complement. However, a C3 (C4) nephritic factor is not always found. In one series, only 2 of 10 patients with C3 glomerulonephritis and monoclonal gammopathy had a C3nef [79]. In another series, none of the 6 patients with MPGN and monoclonal gammopathy demonstrated a C3nef activity but two patients had anti-factor H IgG antibodies [78].

Once the monoclonal protein deposits have been identified in the kidney, the monoclonal protein should be measured in the circulation and the clone responsible should be identified. The monoclonal protein in blood or urine confirms the deposits are monoclonal. It also serves as a marker for treatment response. It is particularly important when there is a biclonal gammopathy to identify the pathologic one for targeting and monitoring. Identification of the clone will allow better and more direct treatment. Many of these clones may be very small, and higher sensitivity techniques such as flow cytometry may be needed. For lymphocytic clones, lymph node biopsy may provide additional information.

Treatment of MGRS

In the past, the risk of therapy-related myelodysplastic syndrome was often considered too high to use cytotoxic therapy for MGRS-related kidney diseases [100]. The one notable exception was AL amyloidosis. Since it is capable of being rapidly fatal, cytotoxic therapy including high-dose chemotherapy was accepted even for patients without multiple myeloma [32, 101, 102]. The same approach, however, was not practiced with the other MGRS-related kidney diseases. In a study of Italian patients with MIDD, patients with multiple myeloma were more likely to receive vincristine–doxorubicin–dexamethasone (VAD) or vincristine–doxorubicin–methylprednisolone (VAMP) than patients without multiple myeloma ($p = 0.007$) [8]. Whether this practice affected the life expectancy of MIDD patients without multiple myeloma was unclear, but the poor renal recovery rate and high recurrence rate after kidney transplant were attributable to inadequate treatment [59, 68]. In diseases with low rate of multiple myeloma such as PGNMID, myeloma therapy was rarely used [74]. Fortunately, the introduction of novel agents in the treatment of multiple myeloma had changed the perspectives. First, concern of myelodysplastic syndrome is much less with novel agents than with alkylators [103]. More importantly, the higher and deeper responses afforded by novel agents have changed the renal outcome of these patients.

Treatment for some of these diseases is covered in greater details in other chapters (Please refer to the respective chapters for details). Instead, this section will cover the principles of treatment. First, as much as possible, treatment should be tailored to each specific clone rather than the kidney disease. In patients without an identifiable clone, one practical approach is to start with cyclophosphamide, bortezomib, and steroids [104]. The use of bortezomib as a frontline agent is preferred over other novel agents due to its rapid response, lack of nephrotoxicity or need for dosage adjustment in renal impairment [105]. Since many of the MGRS-related diseases have low malignant potential, the primary purpose of treatment for most cases (except AL amyloidosis) is preservation of kidney function rather than life [11]. Thus, for patients with advance degree of renal damage with little prospect of renal recovery and no other systemic involvement, and who are not candidates for kidney transplantation, treatment may not be necessary [104]. On the other hand, patients with rapidly declining renal function should be treated aggressively to avoid development of ESRD. Similarly, patients with advance chronic kidney disease or ESRD who are eligible for kidney transplantation should be treated in order to minimize their chances of recurrence after kidney transplantation. One important aspect to keep in mind when treating these patients is the separation between hematologic response and renal response. While renal response is dependent on hematologic response, it is also depended on the severity of the renal damage [35]. Kidneys with advanced damage may not recover despite achievement of complete hematologic response.

Kidney transplantation in the past has been difficult due to the high rate of recurrence and graft loss and ineffective and risky therapies [68]. Adding alkylator therapy to immunosuppression often resulted in overimmunosuppression leading to infection and sepsis. The use of high-dose therapy followed by autologous stem cell transplantation (SCT) has made it possible to perform kidney transplantation in these patients. The achievement of hematologic complete response (CR) either prior to or after kidney transplant has produced satisfactory results in both allograft and patient survival in patients with AL amyloidosis [106]. Similar strategy has been successfully employed in patients with MIDD to prevent recurrence in the kidney allograft [65, 66]. Whether CR is required prior to kidney transplantation remains a question and is dependent on the disease. One consideration is damage to the renal allograft during treatment. Changes in immunosuppression during SCT have resulted in acute rejection of the kidney allograft [107]. Another important aspect is how quickly the disease can recur. In LCDD and PGNMID, recurrence can occur within 3 months of kidney transplantation whereas it is much slower in AL amyloidosis [68, 74, 108]. In diseases with rapid recurrence, achievement of CR should be done prior to kidney transplantation to avoid unnecessary damage to the kidney allograft. With the deep responses novel agents are capable of producing, the question whether SCT is required is valid and pertinent [61, 109–111]. More data are needed for salvage therapy after kidney transplantation before further recommendations can be made.

References

1. Steensma DP, Kyle RA. A history of the kidney in plasma cell disorders. Contrib Nephrol. 2007;153:5–24.
2. Alexanian R, Barlogie B, Dixon D. Renal failure in multiple myeloma. Pathogenesis and prognostic implications. Arch Intern Med. 1990;150 (8):1693–5.
3. Adam Z, et al. [Kidney failure in a patient with chronic B-lymphocytic leukaemia (B-CLL) with underlying cast nephropathy. The value of free

immunoglobulin light chain identification for early diagnosis of this complication]. Vnitrni Lekarstvi. 2011;57(2):214–21.

4. Perez NS, et al. Lymphoplasmacytic lymphoma causing light chain cast nephropathy. Nephrol Dial Transplant Official Publ Eur Dial Transplant Assoc Eur Ren Assoc. 2012;27(1):450–3.

5. Solomon A, Weiss DT, Kattine AA. Nephrotoxic potential of Bence Jones proteins. N Engl J Med. 1991;324(26):1845–51.

6. Kyle RA, Gertz MA. Primary systemic amyloidosis: clinical and laboratory features in 474 cases. Semin Hematol. 1995;32(1):45–59.

7. Nasr SH, et al. Renal monoclonal immunoglobulin deposition disease: a report of 64 patients from a single institution. Clin J Am Soc Nephrol CJASN. 2012;7(2):231–9.

8. Pozzi C, et al. Light chain deposition disease with renal involvement: clinical characteristics and prognostic factors. Am J Kidney Dis Official J National Kidney Found. 2003;42(6):1154–63.

9. Rajkumar SV, Gertz MA, Kyle RA. Primary systemic amyloidosis with delayed progression to multiple myeloma. Cancer. 1998;82(8):1501–5.

10. Kyle RA, et al. Monoclonal gammopathy of undetermined significance (MGUS) and smoldering (asymptomatic) multiple myeloma: IMWG consensus perspectives risk factors for progression and guidelines for monitoring and management. Leukemia. 2010;24(6):1121–7.

11. Leung N, et al. Monoclonal gammopathy of renal significance: when MGUS is no longer undetermined or insignificant. Blood. 2012;120 (22):4292–5.

12. Drayson M, et al. Effects of paraprotein heavy and light chain types and free light chain load on survival in myeloma: an analysis of patients receiving conventional-dose chemotherapy in Medical Research Council UK multiple myeloma trials. Blood. 2006;108(6):2013–9.

13. Merlini G, Bellotti V. Molecular mechanisms of amyloidosis. N Engl J Med. 2003;349(6):583–96 (see comment).

14. Leung N, Nasr SH, Sethi S. How I treat amyloidosis: the importance of accurate diagnosis and amyloid typing. Blood. 2012;120(16):3206–13.

15. Nasr SH., et al. The diagnosis and characteristics of renal heavy-chain and heavy/light-chain amyloidosis and their comparison with renal light-chain amyloidosis. Kidney Int. 2013;83(3):463–70.

16. Mishra S, et al. Human amyloidogenic light chain proteins result in cardiac dysfunction, cell death, and early mortality in zebrafish. Am J Physiol Heart Circ Physiol. 2013;305(1):H95–103.

17. Keeling J, Teng J, Herrera GA. AL-amyloidosis and light-chain deposition disease light chains induce divergent phenotypic transformations of human mesangial cells. Lab Inv J Tech Methods Pathol. 2004;84(10):1322–38.

18. Zeier M, et al. No regression of renal AL amyloid in monoclonal gammopathy after successful autologous blood stem cell transplantation and significant clinical improvement. Nephrol Dial Transplant Official Publ Eur Dial Transplant Assoc Eur Ren Assoc. 2003;18(12):2644–7.

19. Ivanyi B. Frequency of light chain deposition nephropathy relative to renal amyloidosis and Bence Jones cast nephropathy in a necropsy study of patients with myeloma. Arch Pathol Lab Med. 1990;114(9):986–7.

20. Nasr SH, et al. Clinicopathologic correlations in multiple myeloma: a case series of 190 patients with kidney biopsies. Am J Kidney Dis Official J National Kidney Found. 2012;59(6):786–94.

21. Kapadia SB. Multiple myeloma: a clinicopathologic study of 62 consecutively autopsied cases. Medicine. 1980;59(5):380–92.

22. Oshima K, et al. Clinical and pathologic findings in 52 consecutively autopsied cases with multiple myeloma. Am J Hematol. 2001;67(1):1–5.

23. Kourelis TV, et al. Systemic amyloidosis associated with chronic lymphocytic leukemia/small lymphocytic lymphoma. Am J Hematol. 2013;88(5):375–8.

24. Sanchorawala V, et al. AL amyloidosis associated with B-cell lymphoproliferative disorders: frequency and treatment outcomes. Am J Hematol. 2006;81(9):692–5.

25. Leung N, et al. Urinary albumin excretion patterns of patients with cast nephropathy and other monoclonal gammopathy-related kidney diseases. Clin J Am Soc Nephrol CJASN. 2012;7(12):1964–8.

26. Eirin A, et al. Clinical features of patients with immunoglobulin light chain amyloidosis (AL) with vascular-limited deposition in the kidney. Nephrol Dial Transplant Official Publ Eur Dial Transplant Assoc Eur Ren Assoc. 2012;27(3):1097–101.

27. Gertz MA, et al. Clinical outcome of immunoglobulin light chain amyloidosis affecting the kidney. Nephrol Dial Transplant Official Publ Eur Dial Transplant Assoc Eur Ren Assoc. 2009;24(10):3132–7.

28. Lachmann HJ, et al. Misdiagnosis of hereditary amyloidosis as AL (primary) amyloidosis. N Engl J Med. 2002;346(23):1786–91.

29. Kyle RA, et al. A trial of three regimens for primary amyloidosis: colchicine alone, melphalan and prednisone, and melphalan, prednisone, and colchicine. N Engl J Med. 1997;336(17):1202–7 (comment).

30. Cibeira MT, et al. Outcome of AL amyloidosis after high-dose melphalan and autologous stem cell transplantation: long-term results in a series of 421 patients. Blood. 2011;118(16):4346–52.

31. Jaccard A, et al. High-dose melphalan versus melphalan plus dexamethasone for AL amyloidosis. N Engl J Med. 2007;357 (11):1083–93.

32. Palladini G, et al. Treatment with oral melphalan plus dexamethasone produces long-term remissions in AL amyloidosis. Blood. 2007;110 (2):787–8.

33. Leung N, et al. Renal response after high-dose melphalan and stem cell transplantation is a favorable marker in patients with primary systemic amyloidosis. Am J Kidney Dis Official J National Kidney Found. 2005;46(2):270–7.

34. Leung N, et al. A detailed evaluation of the current renal response criteria in AL amyloidosis: is it time for a revision? Haematologica. 2013;98 (6):988–92.

35. Leung N, et al. Severity of baseline proteinuria predicts renal response in immunoglobulin light chain-associated amyloidosis after autologous stem cell transplantation. Clin J Am Soc Nephrol CJASN. 2007;2(3):440–4.
36. Schwartz MM, Lewis EJ. The quarterly case: nephrotic syndrome in a middle-aged man. Ultrastruct Pathol. 1980;1(4):575–82.
37. Bridoux F, et al. Fibrillary glomerulonephritis and immunotactoid (microtubular) glomerulopathy are associated with distinct immunologic features. Kidney Int. 2002;62(5):1764–75.
38. Rosenstock JL, et al. Fibrillary and immunotactoid glomerulonephritis: distinct entities with different clinical and pathologic features. Kidney Int. 2003;63(4):1450–61.
39. Nasr SH, et al. Fibrillary glomerulonephritis: a report of 66 cases from a single institution. Clin J Am Soc Nephrol CJASN. 2011;6(4):775–84.
40. Nasr SH, et al. Immunotactoid glomerulopathy: clinicopathologic and proteomic study. Nephrol Dial Transplant Official Publ Eur Dial Transplant Assoc Eur Ren Assoc. 2012;27(11):4137–46.
41. Ma CX, et al. Acquired Fanconi syndrome is an indolent disorder in the absence of overt multiple myeloma. Blood. 2004;104(1):40–2.
42. Messiaen T, et al. Adult Fanconi syndrome secondary to light chain gammopathy. Clinicopathologic heterogeneity and unusual features in 11 patients. Medicine. 2000;79(3):135–54.
43. Nishida Y, et al. Renal Fanconi syndrome as a cause of chronic kidney disease in patients with monoclonal gammopathy of undetermined significance: partially reversed renal function by high-dose dexamethasone with bortezomib. Leuk Lymphoma. 2012;53(9):1804–6.
44. Kapur U, et al. Expanding the pathologic spectrum of immunoglobulin light chain proximal tubulopathy. Arch Pathol Lab Med. 2007;131 (9):1368–72.
45. Larsen CP, et al. The morphologic spectrum and clinical significance of light chain proximal tubulopathy with and without crystal formation. Mod Pathology Official J US Can Acad Pathol Inc 2011;24(11):1462–9.
46. Herlitz LC, et al. Light chain proximal tubulopathy. Kidney Int. 2009;76 (7):792–7.
47. Sanders PW. Mechanisms of light chain injury along the tubular nephron. J Am Soc Nephrol JASN. 2012;23(11):1777–81.
48. Ramos-Casals M, et al. The cryoglobulinaemias. Lancet. 2012;379 (9813):348–60.
49. Tedeschi A, et al. Cryoglobulinemia. Blood Rev. 2007;21(4):183–200.
50. Saadoun D, et al. Rituximab plus Peg-interferon-alpha/ribavirin compared with Peg-interferon-alpha/ribavirin in hepatitis C-related mixed cryoglobulinemia. Blood. 2010;116(3):326–34;quiz 504–5.
51. Shaikh A, et al. Acute renal failure secondary to severe type I cryoglobulinemia following rituximab therapy for Waldenstrom's macroglobulinemia. Clin Experimental Nephrol. 2008;12(4):292–5.
52. Buxbaum J, Gallo G. Nonamyloidotic monoclonal immunoglobulin deposition disease. Light-chain, heavy-chain, and light- and heavy-chain deposition diseases. Hematol Oncol Clin North Am. 1999;13(6):1235–48.

53. Buxbaum JN, et al. Monoclonal immunoglobulin deposition disease: light chain and light and heavy chain deposition diseases and their relation to light chain amyloidosis. Clinical features, immunopathology, and molecular analysis. Ann Intern Med. 1990;112(6):455–64.
54. Randall RE, et al. Manifestations of systemic light chain deposition. Am J Med. 1976;60(2):293–9.
55. Strom EH, et al. Light chain deposition disease of the kidney. Morphological aspects in 24 patients. Virchows Archiv Int J Pathol. 1994;425(3):271–80.
56. Noel LH, et al. Renal granular monoclonal light chain deposits: morphological aspects in 11 cases. Clin Nephrol. 1984;21(5):263–9.
57. Picken MM, et al. Light chain deposition disease derived from the kappa I light chain subgroup. Biochemical characterization. Am J Pathol. 1989;134(4):749–54.
58. James LC, et al. Beta-edge interactions in a pentadecameric human antibody V kappa domain. J Mol Biol. 2007;367(3):603–8.
59. Heilman RL, et al. Long-term follow-up and response to chemotherapy in patients with light-chain deposition disease. Am J Kidney Dis Official J National Kidney Found. 1992;20(1):34–41.
60. Lin J, et al. Renal monoclonal immunoglobulin deposition disease: the disease spectrum. J Am Soc Nephrol JASN. 2001;12(7):1482–92.
61. Kastritis E, et al. Treatment of light chain deposition disease with bortezomib and dexamethasone. Haematologica. 2009;94(2):300–2.
62. Tovar N, et al. Bortezomib/dexamethasone followed by autologous stem cell transplantation as front line treatment for light-chain deposition disease. Eur J Haematol. 2012;89(4):340–4.
63. Minarik J, et al. Induction treatment of light chain deposition disease with bortezomib: rapid hematological response with persistence of renal involvement. Leuk Lymphoma. 2012;53(2):330–1.
64. Girnius S, et al. Long-term outcome of patients with monoclonal Ig deposition disease treated with high-dose melphalan and stem cell transplantation. Bone Marrow Transplant. 2011;46(1):161–2.
65. Hassoun H, et al. High-dose melphalan and auto-SCT in patients with monoclonal Ig deposition disease. Bone Marrow Transplant. 2008;42(6):405–12.
66. Lorenz EC, et al. Long-term outcome of autologous stem cell transplantation in light chain deposition disease. Nephrol Dial Transplant Official Publ Eur Dial Transplant Assoc Eur Ren Assoc. 2008;23(6):2052–7.
67. Royer B, et al. High dose chemotherapy in light chain or light and heavy chain deposition disease. Kidney Int. 2004;65(2):642–8.
68. Leung N, et al. Long-term outcome of renal transplantation in light-chain deposition disease. Am J Kidney Dis Official J National Kidney Found. 2004;43(1):147–53.
69. Pauekskon P, et al. Monoclonal gammopathy: significance and possible causality in renal disease. Am J Kidney Dis Official J National Kidney Found. 2003;42(1):87–95.

70. Sethi S, Fervenza FC. Membranoproliferative glomerulonephritis–a new look at an old entity. N Engl J Med. 2012;366(12):1119–31.
71. Sethi S, Nester CM, Smith RJ. Membranoproliferative glomerulonephritis and C3 glomerulopathy: resolving the confusion. Kidney Int. 2012;81 (5):434–41.
72. Sethi S, et al. Membranoproliferative glomerulonephritis secondary to monoclonal gammopathy. Clin J Am Soc Nephrology CJASN. 2010;5 (5):770–82.
73. Nasr SH, et al. Proliferative glomerulonephritis with monoclonal IgG deposits. J Am Soc Nephrol JASN. 2009;20(9):2055–64.
74. Nasr SH, et al. Proliferative glomerulonephritis with monoclonal IgG deposits recurs in the allograft. Clinical J Am Soc Nephrol CJASN. 2011;6(1):122–32.
75. Soares SM, et al. A proliferative glomerulonephritis secondary to a monoclonal IgA. Am J Kidney Dis Official J National Kidney Found. 2006;47(2):342–9.
76. Barbour TD, Pickering MC, Cook HT. Recent insights into C3 glomerulopathy. Nephrol Dial Transplant Official Publ Eur Dial Transplant Assoc Eur Ren Assoc. 2013;28(7):1685–93.
77. Sethi S, et al. C3 glomerulonephritis: clinicopathological findings, complement abnormalities, glomerular proteomic profile, treatment, and follow-up. Kidney Int. 2012;82(4):465–73.
78. Bridoux F, et al. Glomerulonephritis with isolated C3 deposits and monoclonal gammopathy: a fortuitous association? Clin J Am Soc Nephrol CJASN. 2011;6(9):2165–74.
79. Zand L, et al. C3 glomerulonephritis associated with monoclonal gammopathy: a case series. Am J Kidney Dis Official J National Kidney Found. 2013;62(3):506–14.
80. Williams DG, Bartlett A, Duffus P. Identification of nephritic factor as an immunoglobulin. Clin Exp Immunol. 1978;33(3):425–9.
81. Davis AE 3rd, et al. Heterogeneity of nephritic factor and its identification as an immunoglobulin. Proc Natl Acad Sci USA. 1977;74(9):3980–3.
82. Tsokos GC, et al. Human polyclonal and monoclonal IgG and IgM complement 3 nephritic factors: evidence for idiotypic commonality. Clin Immunol Immunopathol. 1989;53(1):113–22.
83. Sethi S, et al. Dense deposit disease associated with monoclonal gammopathy of undetermined significance. Am J Kidney Dis. 2010;56 (5):977–82.
84. Ofran Y, Elinav E. POEMS syndrome: failure of newly suggested diagnostic criteria to anticipate the development of the syndrome. Am J Hematol. 2005;79(4):316–8.
85. Dispenzieri A. POEMS syndrome: update on diagnosis, risk-stratification, and management. Am J Hematol. 2012;87(8):804–14.
86. Clapp AJ, et al. Imaging evidence for renomegaly in patients with POEMS syndrome. Acad Radiol. 2011;18(10):1241–4.
87. Nakamoto Y, et al. A spectrum of clinicopathological features of nephropathy associated with POEMS syndrome. Nephrol Dial Transplant

Official Publ Eur Dial Transplant Assoc Eur Ren Assoc. 1999;14 (10):2370–8.

88. Navis GJ, et al. Renal disease in POEMS syndrome: report on a case and review of the literature. Nephrol Dial Transplant Official Publ Eur Dial Transplant Assoc Eur Ren Assoc. 1994;9(10):1477–81.

89. Chazot C, et al. Crow-Fukase disease/POEMS syndrome presenting with severe microangiopathic involvement of the kidney. Nephrol Dial Transplant Official Publ Eur Dial Transplant Assoc Eur Ren Assoc. 1994;9(12):1800–2.

90. Higashi AY, et al. Serial renal biopsy findings in a case of POEMS syndrome with recurrent acute renal failure. Clin Experimental Nephrol. 2012;16(1):173–9.

91. Soubrier M, et al. Growth factors and proinflammatory cytokines in the renal involvement of POEMS syndrome. Am J Kidney Dis Official J National Kidney Found. 1999;34(4):633–8.

92. Sprangers B, Kuypers DR. Recurrence of glomerulonephritis after renal transplantation. Transplant Rev. 2013;27(4):126–34.

93. Gera M, et al. Recurrence of ANCA-associated vasculitis following renal transplantation in the modern era of immunosupression. Kidney Int. 2007;71(12):1296–301.

94. Short AK, et al. Recurrence of light chain nephropathy in a renal allograft. A case report and review of the literature. Am J Nephrol. 2001;21(3):237–40.

95. Czarnecki PG, et al. Long-term outcome of kidney transplantation in patients with fibrillary glomerulonephritis or monoclonal gammopathy with fibrillary deposits. Kidney Int. 2009;75(4):420–7.

96. Lorenz EC, et al. Recurrent membranoproliferative glomerulonephritis after kidney transplantation. Kidney Int. 2010;77(8):721–8.

97. Kyle RA, et al. Prevalence of monoclonal gammopathy of undetermined significance. N Engl J Med. 2006;354(13):1362–9.

98. Swaminathan S, et al. Changing incidence of glomerular disease in Olmsted County, Minnesota: a 30-year renal biopsy study. Clin J Am Soc Nephrol CJASN. 2006;1(3):483–7.

99. Vrana JA, et al. Classification of amyloidosis by laser microdissection and mass spectrometry-based proteomic analysis in clinical biopsy specimens. Blood. 2009;114(24):4957–9.

100. Cuzick J, et al. A comparison of the incidence of the myelodysplastic syndrome and acute myeloid leukaemia following melphalan and cyclophosphamide treatment for myelomatosis. A report to the Medical Research Council's working party on leukaemia in adults. Br J Cancer. 1987;55(5):523–9.

101. Kyle RA, Greipp PR. Primary systemic amyloidosis: comparison of melphalan and prednisone versus placebo. Blood. 1978;52(4):818–27.

102. Skinner M, et al. High-dose melphalan and autologous stem-cell transplantation in patients with AL amyloidosis: an 8-year study. Ann Intern Med. 2004;140(2):85–93.

103. Rajkumar SV. Treatment of multiple myeloma. Nature reviews. Clinical oncology. 2011;8(8):479–91.

104. Fermand JP, et al. How I treat monoclonal gammopathy of renal significance (MGRS). Blood. 2013;122(22):3583–90.
105. Chanan-Khan AA, et al. Activity and safety of bortezomib in multiple myeloma patients with advanced renal failure: a multicenter retrospective study. Blood. 2007;109(6):2604–6.
106. Herrmann SM, et al. Long-term outcomes of patients with light chain amyloidosis (AL) after renal transplantation with or without stem cell transplantation. Nephrol Dial Transplant Official Publ Eur Dial Transplant Assoc Eur Ren Assoc. 2011;26(6):2032–6.
107. Leung N, et al. Acute cellular rejection in a renal allograft immediately following leukocyte engraftment after auto-SCT. Bone Marrow Transplant. 2009;43(4):345–6.
108. Pinney JH, et al. Renal transplantation in systemic amyloidosis-importance of amyloid fibril type and precursor protein abundance. Am J Transplant Official J Am Soc Transplant Am Soc Transplant Surg. 2013;13(2):433–41.
109. Kastritis E, et al. Treatment of light chain (AL) amyloidosis with the combination of bortezomib and dexamethasone. Haematologica. 2007;92 (10):1351–8.
110. Mikhael JR, et al. Cyclophosphamide-bortezomib-dexamethasone (CyBorD) produces rapid and complete hematologic response in patients with AL amyloidosis. Blood. 2012;119(19):4391–4.
111. Wechalekar AD, et al. Safety and efficacy of risk-adapted cyclophosphamide, thalidomide, and dexamethasone in systemic AL amyloidosis. Blood. 2007;109(2):457–64.

Index

Note: Page numbers followed by *'f'* and *'t'* refer to figures and tables, respectively

© Springer Science+Business Media New York 2017
T.M. Zimmerman and S.K. Kumar (eds.),
Biology and Management of Unusual Plasma Cell Dyscrasias,
DOI 10.1007/978-1-4419-6848-7

Printed in the United States
By Bookmasters